QUALITY
MANAGEMENT
REVIEW

QUALITY MANAGEMENT REVIEW

Steven B. Dowd, Ed.D., RT(R)(QM)(M)(MR)(CT)CPHQ
Associate Professor
Program Director Radiography Program
University of Alabama at Birmingham
Birmingham, Alabama

Elwin R. Tilson, Ed.D., RT(R)(QM)(M)(CT)
Professor of Radiologic Technologist
Armstrong State College
Savannah, Georgia

Richard R. Carlton, M.S., R.T.(R)FAERS
Assistant Professor of Radiologic Sciences
Arkansas State University
State University, Arkansas

DELMAR

™

THOMSON LEARNING   Australia   Canada   Mexico   Singapore   Spain   United Kingdom   United States

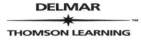

Quality Review Management

by Stephen B. Dowd, Elwin R. Tilson, Richard R. Carlton

Business Unit Director:
William Brottmiller

Executive Marketing Manager:
Dawn F. Gerrain

Production Coordinator:
Catherine Ciardullo

Acquisitions Editor:
Candice Janco

Executive Editor:
Cathy L. Esperti

Art/Design Coordinator:
Jay Purcell

Editorial Assistant:
Maria D'Angelico

Project Editor
Jim Zayicek

Library of Congress Cataloging-in-Publication Data
ISBN-07668-1258-8

Contents

Preface

USING THIS TEXT TO THE BEST ADVANTAGE

This text is designed for radiographers wishing to take the Advanced Certification Examination in Quality Management (QM) offered by the American Registry of Radiologic Technologists (ARRT). It could be used in a number of other settings where quality management is taught as well. In addition to study questions, Chapter 1 of *Quality Management Review* contains a detailed listing of "Knowledge Points"–facts relevant to the QM exam, that would be useful for a class in quality improvement/management.

Each chapter includes a brief overview of the material or questions similar in format and content to those on the ARRT examination. We have not attempted to completely mirror the ARRT examination as we believe a book of this type must have both educational and assessment components. Thus, some of the questions attempt to teach as well as assess by using formats such as True/False or All of the Above.

The basic formula of the book is to have at least three times as many questions as each section of the examination, although some *sub*sections will have more; some less. This essentially correlates with the breadth of coverage needed, depending on the subject matter.

Each chapter of questions has annotated answers at the end that indicate why the choice is correct, as well as why the distractors (the incorrect choices) are incorrect. We have made an attempt to explain the answers for optimal review. There also is one final post-test matching the examination to help gauge progress.

ACKNOWLEDGMENTS
Steven B. Dowd

Thanks to my wife, Lisa and son, Josh for helping me out through my various certification endeavors (including obsessing over my expected score on the QM exam) and the writing of this book. Also, thanks to Ann Steves and Randal Robertson for their professional support during the writing of this book and in my teaching.

Elwin R. Tilson

I would like to acknowledge Dr. Sharyn Gibson, Gloria Strickland, Debbie Lamb, and Sharon Gillard-Smith—my professional colleagues who have nurtured me, taught me, inspired me, and worked with me over the years. I also owe a great debt to my students who have inspired me by always asking "Why?". Finally, this book would never been published without the hard work of Candice Janco and Marie D'Angelico, both of Delmar Thomson Learning. Thank you all!

Richard B. Carlton

A professional life requires a wide range of support to be successful. The extent to which mine has succeeded recently is in great measure due to a great dean, chair, and our faculty at Arkansas State. Thanks to Susan Hanrahan, Ray Winters, Lyn Hubbard, Jeannean Rollins, Tracy White, and Lynn Carlton (who shares both my professional and personal life).

ABOUT THE AUTHORS

Dr. Steven B. Dowd is Program Director and Associate Professor for the B.S. Radiologic Sciences program at University of Alabama at Birmingham, as well as a faculty member in both the nuclear medicine technology and radiation therapy programs. A member of the graduate faculty, he also serves on dissertation committees in the UAB School of Nursing. He has 20 years of experience teaching and practicing radiography and advanced imaging.

A graduate of Nova Southeastern University, the University of Illinois-Springfield, Regent's College, and Parkland College, his research interests include Gerontology, Quality Management, Radiation Protection, and Effective Teaching, especially the teaching/learning environment for adult learners and the development of effective teaching materials. He is the author or coauthor of seven books, 100 peer-reviewed articles, and 300 total articles in the health sciences literature. He is certified in a number of areas including radiography, quality management, mammography, magnetic resonance imaging, and computed tomography.

Dr. Elwin R. Tilson is Professor and Clinical Coordinator of Radiologic Sciences at Armstrong Atlantic State University in Savannah, GA. Dr. Tilson completed his radiography education in the U.S. Army in 1969, earned a bachelor of science degree in radiologic technology from Arizona State University in 1975, a master of science degree in allied health education from San Francisco State University in 1978, and a doctorate with an emphasis in education technology from the University of Georgia in 1986.

Dr. Tilson has extensive experience in general radiography, trauma radiography, computed tomography, neuroradiology, educational administration, and quality computed tomography management. He is certified in radiography, mammography, and quality management, and is the coauthor of a radiation biology text, a quality management computer program, and numerous articles.

Richard R. Carlton is an Assistant Professor of Radiologic Sciences, Arkansas State University. Rick is a Charter Fellow of the Association of Educators in Radiologic Sciences, holds a master's degree from National Louis University, a bachelor's degree from the University of Health Sciences/The Chicago Medical School, and a pair of associate degrees from Illinois Central College.

Rick has taught radiography for 23 years and speaks regularly throughout the world. He has authored 16 books and founded two journals.

Rick is currently the director of the Center for Medical Imaging in Bioanthropology at Arkansas State, where he is involved in x-raying mummies all over the world. For more information on his work, visit him online at www.clt.astate. edu/RadSci/cmib.htm.

Studying for the QM Registry

One of the most important challenges in studying for the QM registry is to figure out how to learn the broad mass of material required for the test. There are many usable sources, but no single source is comprehensive. We suggest following several rules:

Rule 1: Know your physics and imaging.

Rule 2: Do not rely on one source.

Rule 3: Make a notebook that contains all the sources you have compiled.

Rule 4: Drill-and-review often.

Rule 5: Make certain you ***understand*** QI/QM concepts.

RECOMMENDED REFERENCES

Diagnostic Imaging

Papp, J. *Quality Management in the Imaging Sciences* (Mosby-Yearbook, 1998) is currently the main resource for QM for radiography.

This book is an excellent overview of quality control (Chapters 2–11) in diagnostic imaging. The author has an excellent command of radiographic equipment and accessories.

Use this book for an overview of QC in diagnostic radiology. Try other sources for actual drill-and-review, most non-radiology regulations and accreditation guidelines, and understanding QM as an overall concept.

Physics

There are a number of books that provide information on physics for the radiologic sciences.

Mammography

There is no substitute for actually reading the American College of Radiology (ACR) manual. However, Papp provides a good start for QC in mammography in *Quality Management in the Imaging Sciences.*

Be sure to develop some method for distinguishing between QC in mammography and general radiography because tolerances, etc. are not exactly the same.

Film Processing

The best resource for film processing is Haus and Jaskulski's *The Basics of Film Processing in Medical Imaging* (Medical Physics Publishing, 1997), although McKinney's *Radiographic Processing and Quality Control* (initially Lippincott, republished in 1997 through another company) runs a close second. The material in Haus and Jaskulski particularly on hard-to-find information such as the make-up and operation of densitometers, flooded replenishment, etc. is extremely valuable in test preparation.

Note: The proper term $D_{LOG}E$ curve is used throughout this book to describe what is also known as a Hurter and Driffield (H&D) curve, characteristic curve, sensitometric curve, or film average gradient (gamma) curve.

Government Regulations and Accreditation Guidelines

There is again no substitute for getting original copies of the government documents, such as CFR 1910.1030 (bloodborne pathogens), NCRP 99 and 105, and at least reviewing the JCAHO guide. Some of these are available on the Internet, and public domain documents can be photocopied at your local medical library.

In addition, there is a good chapter on the Safe Medical Devices Act in Ann Obergfell's law book, *Law and Ethics in Diagnostic Imaging and Therapeutic Radiology* (WB Saunders, 1995).

Another great source for understanding definitions in the quality arena is Timmreck's *Health Services Cyclopedic Dictionary*, 3rd ed., (Boston, Jones, & Bartlett, 1997). This one may be available in the reference section of your library. If not, you may want to try an interlibrary loan. If you have trouble understanding things like the difference between "effectiveness" and "efficacy" (like we do), then this book (along with relevant pages from the JCAHO guide) will help you tremendously.

QM/QI

Adams & Aurora's book contains especially good test items and diagrams relating to the QM process. Chapter 6 of Steve Hiss' book, *Introduction to Health Care Delivery and Radiology Administration* (WB Saunders, 1997) has a good introduction to QI. Tilson & Dowd's article, "The benefits of using CQI/TQM data" in *Radiologic Technology*, Vol. 67, no. 6, 1996:

pages 533–537, is also useful. Other good QM philosophy and systems sources are Lauglin & Kaluzny's *Continuous Quality Improvement in Health Care* (Aspen, 1994). The National Association for Healthcare Quality (NAHQ) publishes the *Guide to Quality Management,* 8th ed. (1998), which is written for their Certified Professional in Healthcare Quality (CPHQ) exam.

The American Society of Radiologic Technologists (ASRT) also sells two good homestudies on QM by Rebecca Lam that we think would help anyone needing to learn the basics of QM.

Statistics

The statistical concepts on the QM registry are basic, but you must know them well. Don't expect simple questions like "What is the mean?"; you must instead know how to calculate the mean and what it is used for. Do your best to find a good statistics book that makes sense to you. Nursing statistics books tend to give examples that are closest to radiography; e.g., Burns & Grove, *The Practice of Nursing Research: Conduct, Critique, and Utilization* (WB Saunders, 2001).

Drill-and-Review

There are two good drill-and-review programs: one distributed by Corectec of Athens, Georgia, and one through Educational Software Concepts Inc. (ESC), by Elwin Tilson and Steven Dowd. The ESC disk is about $30 and contains over 600 questions with detailed annotated answers. You can drill-and-review in specific sections and take multiple mock registries. The Corectec disk is about $99 and contains one well-designed mock registry.

BASIC MATERIAL YOU NEED TO KNOW

Although it is not recommended to simply memorize material for this, or any other certification exam, here are some useful starting points with basic things you should know before moving on to critical thinking about the material in the examination. Alternately, you can look upon them as "study notes" to be used in the same fashion as if you had taken a formal class– they contain the "bare bones" of the material, but not enough for in-depth understanding.

This section contains lists of **knowledge points** from some of the main reference documents. This is, of course, material from several books and cannot be considered complete in its description. When possible, key points from governmental regulations have been cited in their entirety, or summarized.

NCRP #105 (Sections 1, 2, 6, 7, 8)
Main source for radiation protection information for the examination

KNOWLEDGE POINT 1.1:
The "Shalls" and "Shoulds"

- *shall*–recommendation that is necessary or essential to meet the currently accepted standards of protection

- *should*–an advisory recommendation that is to be applied when practicable

The specific shalls and shoulds are contained behind each memorization point.

KNOWLEDGE POINT 1.2:
Radiation Units

- Exposure–Roentgen (R) and columb per kilogram (c/kg)
- Absorbed dose–gray (Gy) and rad (gray is also defined as the unit of kerma)
- Dose equivalent–Sievert (Sv) or rem
- Activity–Becquerel and Curie

KNOWLEDGE POINT 1.3:
Sources of Radiation

- Naturally occurring (background) radiation–cosmic and terrestrial
- Patient doses–Typical exposures; U.S. average (39 mrem or 0.39 mSv)
- Occupational exposure

KNOWLEDGE POINT 1.4:
Sources of Radiation Exposure in the Medical Environment

- Radioactive materials
- Half-life (50%) of original intensity remains after each; 1/10 of 1% (0.1%) of the original number after 10 half-lives)
- Alpha, beta, and gamma radiations
- Sealed and unsealed sources (e.g., brachytherapy)
- Types of radiation-producing equipment–Diagnostic, therapeutic

KNOWLEDGE POINT 1.5:

Basic Principles of Radiation Protection

Time, Distance, Shielding

- Technologists *should* stand as far away as possible (at least two meters) from the x-ray tube and patient. Always use appropriate shielding or be out of the room when possible.

Survey Meters

- Geigen-Muller (GM) counter (qualitative measurements only), portable scintillation counters, and ionization chambers are most often used.

- Individuals involved in the handling of radioactive materials *shall* be competent in the use of survey meters.

- The response of radiation detection instruments *shall* be checked periodically using an appropriate radiation source.

- The radiation safety officer (RSO) *should* be consulted prior to the procurement of survey meters.

- Personnel dosimeters–Types, where worn, minimal exposures

- The site where the dosimeter is worn *should* be documented in the records.

KNOWLEDGE POINT 1.6:
Radioactive Materials Labels, Signs, and Warning Lights

Shoulds

- Use contamination control measures for radioactive materials.
- Restrict use to authorized locations.
- Do not allow in areas where its presence can be an unsuspected source of radiation exposure to the patient.
- Use warning signs.
- Display the recognized magenta radiation symbol on a yellow background.
- Follow explicitly any instructions given on the signs.

Shalls

- Employees shall be given appropriate training and safety instruction by a qualified individual.
- Follow all such instructions and directions.

KNOWLEDGE POINT 1.7:
Acquisition, Storage, and Disposition of Radioactive Materials

Shoulds

- Obtain approved purchase orders in advance from RSO or designee.
- Maintain inventory.

- Store materials in secured locked area.

- Inform all users of records to be kept and procedures to be followed in preparing and disposing radioactive waste.

- Keep users and potentially involved ancillary personnel aware of institutional emergency procedures.

- Supervise all shipments leaving the facility.

Shalls

- Allow only authorized users to order and receive radionuclides.

- Do not exceed individual authorizations for type and amount of radionuclides.

- Have materials delivered to a designated receiving area.

- Provide a designated receiving site for night and weekend deliveries (*should* be accompanied by guard to this site; guard *should* be able to inspect package and call RSO, if needed).

- No food allowed in refrigerator with radioactive materials.

- No eating, drinking, or smoking permitted.

KNOWLEDGE POINT 1.8:
Radioactive Waste Management
Shoulds

- Consult RSO and policy manual before making decisions on disposal of materials.

- Ensure RSO supervises packaging of waste for shipment.

- Segregate radioactive and infectious wastes from ordinary trash.

- Inspect unwanted materials such as tissue or infectious material for decay prior to storage.

Shalls

- Appropriately package and manage waste.

- Plan releases to environment under the supervision of RSO.

- Perform releases in accordance with federal, state, and local regulations.

- Record and maintain releases to sewer.

- Sterilize infectious and radioactive waste before disposal.

KNOWLEDGE POINT 1.9:

Diagnostic Radiographers

This is probably the most important section to know since it directly relates to QA/QC/Radiation Protection in diagnostic radiology.

Shoulds

- Achieve familiarity with equipment and operating procedures.

- Periodically consult RSO, physicist, radiologist, or chief technologist to ensure proper radiation safety practices are being followed.

- Become familiar with CDRH regulations for equipment manufacturing.

- Be aware of approximate personnel radiation exposure.

- Direct beam to achieve minimal exposure to all and to obtain optimal image quality.

- Be aware of shielding and use equipment accordingly.

- Use beam centering when available and carefully collimate to area of clinical interest.

- Stand as far away as practical from tube housing.

- Avoid holding patients routinely.

- Hold patients only when restraining or positioning devices are inadequate.

- Provide lead aprons and gloves and achieve positioning so that no body part is exposed to beam.

- Prohibit pregnant women or individuals under 18 from holding patients.

- Review and implement guidelines by the radiation safety committee.

- Assure that walls are designed to protect and operators remain protected during exposure.

- Assure that exposure switches cannot energize the tube when exposing radiographer is outside shielded areas.

- Dosimeter is normally worn at waist or collar level *outside of aprons.*

- Never allow dose equivalent to a fetus to exceed 0.5 mSv (50 mrem) per month.

- In fluoroscopy, set safety standards, including placement of bucky slot cover, maximum distance to source, use of lead gloves and lead drape, and room inspection guidelines by RSO.

- When using mobile equipment, set safety standards, including a check to see if the cord is long enough for operator to stand 2m from source (patient). (cord may be short if the console is used for protection), ensure operator is cognizant of orientation of the beam with respect to others, and maximize SSD to reduce patient exposure.

- In dental, set safety standards to include proper location of exposure so that operator can stand behind barrier, ensure operator does not hold film or tube, and that a proper beam limiting device is used.

Shalls

- Have an orientation program on radiation safety for newly employed technologists and a continuing education program to review the rules and regulations.

- Make technologists aware of the approximate amount of radiation received by their patients during each radiographic procedure used in their facility.

- Never allow beam size to exceed size of image receptor for radiographic and fluoroscopic procedures.

- Wear a lead apron in fluoroscopy.

NCRP #99
Main source for quality assurance programs in radiology (Sections 1, 6, 7)

KNOWLEDGE POINT 2.1:
Definition of QA

- Quality assurance is a comprehensive concept that comprises all practices instituted by the imaging physician to ensure that:

  1. every imaging procedure is necessary and appropriate to the clinical problem at hand.

  2. the images generated contain information critical to the solution of that problem.

  3. the recorded information is correctly interpreted and made available in a timely fashion to the patient's physician.

  4. the examination results in the lowest possible radiation exposure, cost, and inconvenience to the patient consistent with objective.

KNOWLEDGE POINT 2.2:
Storage, Darkroom, and Processing Conditions

- Photographic materials should be stored at less than 24°C (75°F), preferably 15–21°C (60–70°F); humidity 40–60%. Keep materials from fumes and pressure.

- Darkroom should be adequately illuminated, painted white or light colors, with an appropriate temperature and humidity (40–60%) and lead in walls.

● Most darkrooms will fog film; small amounts of dark-room fog increase the apparent speed and density of the film, but decrease contrast.

● When testing for darkroom fog:

   1. Use the fastest film normally handled in darkrooms, or the fastest of each type.

   2. Make a visible light exposure using a step wedge or densitometer.

   3. Ideally, show less than 0.05 OD increase in middle density region (1.2 OD) with a two-minute expo-sure; less than 0.05 OD increase with one-minute exposure is acceptable.

   4. *Do not* test using unexposed film.

   5. Testing must be done every six months.

KNOWLEDGE POINT 2.3:

Processor Quality Control

● Best method–freshly exposed sensitometric strip read with densitometer.

● pH specific gravity, or bromide concentration methods are not as valid.

● Some basic parameters–should be same film as routinely used, recently exposed to light, and eliminate as many variables as possible.

● Measure:

   1. Base + fog (B + F)

   2. Mid-density or speed point [1.0 + (B + F)]

3. Average gradient (slope of straight line of $D_{LOG}E$ curve)

LOG exposure $(2.50 + B + F) - (0.25 + B + F)$.

Sometimes referred to as the D.D.

Upper and lower control limits

Speed point and average gradient $= \pm0.10$

$B + F = \pm0.05$

Note: These numbers can vary and this does not affect the validity of the data as long as they are consistent throughout the results being compared.

- Isolate an emulsion batch of film sufficient to last at least one month, and you must do a "crossover" (where the speed point and D.D. of the new emulsion batch is compared to the old emulsion batch and the points "reset" on the chart.

- Some other basic parameters may include:

    1. Assign one individual to the program.

    2. Process strips same way each time, and at the same time each day.

    3. Clean and maintain equipment.

KNOWLEDGE POINT 2.4:

Fixer/Archival Quality

- Follow manufacturer's recommendations for flow, etc.

- For archival purposes, staining should be prevented for at least 10 years; preferably 20–25 years.

- Fixer retention test must be done at least every six months, preferably every three.

- Less than $2\mu g/cm^2$ thiosulfate ion (fixer) should remain in film after washing.

KNOWLEDGE POINT 2.5:

Time/Temperature/Rate

- Transport time is measured using a stop watch (on installation and yearly thereafter).

- Developer temperature should be maintained within $\pm0.3°C$ ($0.5°F$); fixer within $\pm3°C$ ($5°F$).

- *Never use a mercury thermometer.*

KNOWLEDGE POINT 2.6:

Flow Rate, Replenishment, and Filters

- Flow rate should be checked daily.

- Replenishment rate must be kept accurate (check calibration of meters quarterly).

- Filters should not allow particles larger than 25 µm to pass.

KNOWLEDGE POINT 2.7:

Filtration

- Increases in the half-valve layer (HVL) tend to lower patient exposure; most noticeable with larger patients (with thicker body parts).

- When measuring HVL, use a dosimeter and sheets of type 1100 aluminum; measure annually as well as when tubes are replaced/serviced, or when collimator is serviced.

KNOWLEDGE POINT 2.8:

Light Field/Collimation

- Light field must be accurate; allow collimation to smaller size than film, even with positive beam limitation (PBL).

- There are a number of ways to measure, including nine coins or paper clips.

- Follow allowances:

  - ±2% of source-to-image receptor distance (SID) in collimator light-to-x-ray field total misalignment.

  - Center of field aligned to center of image ±2% of SID.

  - SID indicator accurate ±2%.

  - Manual collimation x-y scale indicators accurate ±2% of SID.

  - PBL, length or width of x-ray field, cannot differ by more than ±3% of SID compared to image dimension; sum of absolute values of both must not be more than ±4%.

KNOWLEDGE POINT 2.9:

Beam and Bucky Perpendicularity

- Beam and bucky must be centered and perpendicular (avoid grid cut-off).

- Procedure: Radiograph a homogeneous phantom with lead strips in middle to mark center of beam. Lead strips must be in center of beam, and film must be uniform within ±0.10 OD side-to-side (preferably anode-to-cathode axis).

KNOWLEDGE POINT 2.10:
Focal Spot Size

- Acceptance testing may not be a worthwhile regular QA check.

- If using NEMA standards, a slit camera is needed.

KNOWLEDGE POINT 2.11:
Tube Rating Charts

- Tube heat sensor should provide a warning (or exposure terminator) when anode heat reaches 75% of maximum.

- Four types of charts used are single exposure, anode thermal and fluoroscopic, housing cooling charts, and angiographic and cine rating charts.

KNOWLEDGE POINT 2.12:
kVp

- One of most important factors that affects quality of beam, patient exposure, and contrast and density of film.

- Invasive or noninvasive testing

- Noninvasive-Ardran and Crooks cassette ±3 kVp

- New electronic devices accurate ±2% and reproducible ± 0.5 kVp

KNOWLEDGE POINT 2.13:

Exposure Timers

- Tools–spin top (motorized or non-motorized); electronic timing device to measure number of pulses or time

- 3-phase generators ±5% for times in excess of minimum exposure time; one dot variance allowed on single phase at 1/5 and 1/10 seconds and none at 1/20 and 1/30 seconds

- Measure at least annually, when problems occur with light or dark films, and when repair has occurred on generator.

KNOWLEDGE POINT 2.14:

Exposure per Unit of Tube Current and Time

- Measurement of $\mu C/kg^1$ mAs–difficult to measure mAs directly.

- Measure exposure at fixed kVp and mAs; set geometrical conditions.

- Divide the exposure by the mAs (using the "old units"). Many places measure the mR/mAs.

- Exposure should be maintained ±10% at 80 kVp for rooms using the same types of generators, tubes, and tables. If not, each unit needs a different technique chart.

- Measure at least annually.

KNOWLEDGE POINT 2.15:

Linearity and Reproducibility

● *Linearity*–selecting various mA and timer stations that produce the same mAs; producing radiographs of similar density.

▪ Measure using a dosimeter and a fixed kVp (may later vary kVp for additional measurements; keep fixed at first).

▪ ±10% between adjacent mA stations (with six stations, may vary as much as 50%); but *should* be able to maintain across entire generator at ±10%.

● *Reproducibility*–make an exposure; change kVp, mA, and exposure time; go back to original values; have similar output; make three exposures (not three consecutive exposures using same technique and same output without resetting the factors).

▪ ±5% variation from average allowance

▪ Measure at least annually and for troubleshooting.

KNOWLEDGE POINT 2.16:

Phototimers

● Maximum possible exposure cannot exceed 600 mAs.

● Phototimer evaluation at various mA stations should be ±10%.

● If using a homogeneous phantom, OD should be about 1.2, with a variance of ±0.030; film density variations cannot exceed ±0.20 OD.

● Reproducibility should be ±5% of average exposure.

- Density controls should represent equal percentage changes.

KNOWLEDGE POINT 2.17:

Grids

- *Uniformity*–evaluated using homogeneous phantom, 1.2 OD.

    - Dark or light areas are grounds for rejection.

    - No grid lines allowed for bucky.

    - Density should not vary more than ±0.10 OD perpendicular to anode-cathode axis.

    - Must be tested prior to use and annually thereafter (grid cassettes and stationary grids must be tested every six months).

- *Alignment*–same as for film.

KNOWLEDGE POINT 2.18:

Cassettes, Screens, and Films

- Requires proper spectral matching (matching film sensitivity to intensifying screen phosphor emission).

- Densities of similar screens and films should be within ±0.05 OD. If not, take out of service or place in isolated use.

- Must have screen-film contact

- Use wire mesh test. (Wait 15 minutes to expose after loading.)

- Check prior to use, and at least annually thereafter, as well as in response to problems.

- Screen cleaning–check at least every six months.

KNOWLEDGE POINT 2.19:
Patient Equivalent Phantom

- Last quality control check in a room, troubleshooting problems, etc.
- Measure with exposure.
- Center density equals 1.20 ±0.15 OD.
- Similar densities are perpendicular and parallel to anode-cathode axis.
- Exposure should range from 100–150 µC kg^{-1} (400–600 mR).

ACR Manual (Mammography Criteria)

KNOWLEDGE POINT 3.1:
Mammography Tests and Their Parameters

- Daily Tests
  - Darkroom cleanliness: Damp wipe counter tops, wipe feed trays, and damp mop floor
  - Processor quality control: M.D. & D.D. ± 0.15 and B+F ± 0.03
- Weekly Tests
  - Screen cleanliness: Clean screens with approved cleaning agent
  - Illuminators (viewboxes) and viewing conditions: Clean plastic/glass covers, assure units provide luminance of 3,500 nit

- Monthly Tests

  - Phantom images: Must see 4 fibers, 3 specks, and 3 masses. D.D. of 0.40 ± 0.05

  - Visual checklist: Mechanical integrity of locks, SID, etc.

- Quarterly Tests

  - Repeat analysis: Less than 2% repeat rate ideal but may not exceed 5%

  - Fixer retention: Should not exceed Stain #2 (Kodak) which equals 0.05 g/m^2

- Semiannual Tests:

  - Darkroom fog: +0.05

  - Screen-film contact: Large areas unacceptable (greater than 1 cm) and up to 5 small areas (less than 1 cm) acceptable

  - Compressor: Power drive should be 25–40 pounds and manual drive between 25 and 40 pounds.

- Miscellaneous Tests

  - Replace illuminator bulbs every 18–24 months.

KNOWLEDGE POINT 3.2:

Physicist Performed Tests (Annual Basis)

- Average glandular dose
- Artifact evaluation
- Automatic exposure control performance assessment
- Automatic exposure control reproducibility
- Breast entrance exposure
- Collimation assessment

- Focal spot size
- Half-value layer
- Image quality evaluation
- kVp accuracy
- kVp reproducibility
- Uniformity of screen speed
- Unit Assembly inspection

OSHA Guidelines (CFR 1910.1030)

KNOWLEDGE POINT 4.1:

Some Basic Definitions

- *Engineering Controls*–controls that isolate or remove the bloodborne pathogen hazard from the workplace.

- *Exposure incident*–a specific eye, mouth, other mucous membrane, non-intact skin, or parenteral contact with blood or other potentially infectious material that results from performance of an employee's duties.

- *Occupational exposure*–reasonably anticipated skin, eye, mucous membrane, or parenteral contact with blood or other potentially infectious materials that may result from the performance of an employee's duties.

- *Personal protective equipment*–specialized clothing or equipment worn by an employee for protection against a hazard (normal clothing is not included).

- *Work practice controls*–used to reduce the likelihood for exposure by altering the manner in which a task is performed.

KNOWLEDGE POINT 4.2:

What Must the Employer Do?

- Maintain an Exposure Control Plan.

- Determine probability of exposure.

- Institute engineering and work practice controls and ensure employees follow these.

- Provide and maintain personal protective equipment if there is potential for occupational exposure.

- Regulate housekeeping including equipment and regulated waste.

- Make the HBV vaccine available to employees with potential for exposure, at little or no cost, in a reasonable time and place.

- Have a plan for post-exposure evaluation and follow-up.

- Use appropriate labels and signs.

- Provide information and training to employees.

- Maintain appropriate records (e.g., training, HBV vaccination records), and maintain their confidentiality.

KNOWLEDGE POINT 4.3:

Basic Facts About MSDS

- Typically used to comply with OSHA's Hazard Communication Standard, 29 CFR 1910.1200.

- A number of methods are used to communicate vital information. Hazards may be ranked numerically or given descriptively. Possible sections include:

  Section 1   Manufacturer's name, address, etc.

  Section 2   Hazardous Ingredients/Identity–including chemical names

Section 3   Physical and Chemical Characteristics–boiling point, solubility and reactivity in water, appearance and odor melting point

Section 4   Fire and Explosion Date–including flash point, special fire fighting procedures, unusual first and explosion hazards

Section 5   Physical Hazards or Reactivity data–stability, etc.

Section 6   Health Hazards–acute and chronic, medical conditions aggravated by exposure, whether it is a known carcinogen, routes of entry, emergency and first aid procedures

Section 7   Special Precautions and Spill/Leak Procedures

Section 8   Special Protection Information–respiratory protection, gloves, other required clothing

- To obtain additional information, check many manufacturers' Web pages on the Internet, which are often listed on the product.

KNOWLEDGE POINT 4.4:
Basic Facts About the Safe Medical Devices Act of 1991 (SMDA)

- The SMDA acts as a reporting mechanism for unsafe devices. Two major components are adverse event reporting and medical device tracking.

- Use Form 3500 for voluntary reporting and 3500A for mandatory reporting.

- Report to FDA via an 800 number if necessary. (Previous regulations allowed an employee to report to

the employer; now the employee can be fined several
thousand dollars for failure to report).

- An unsafe device is one that causes illness, injury, or
death to a patient.

- User facilities are hospitals, nursing homes, outpatient
treatment centers, and ambulatory surgical facilities.
Physician offices and group practices are affected
through the tracking rule.

KNOWLEDGE POINT 4.5:

Aggregate Data JCAHO Indicators

- Appropriateness of care–is the care necessary?

- Continuity of care–how is care coordinated among
practitioners and organizations?

- Effectiveness of care–what is the level of benefit of care
(under ordinary circumstances, average practitioners,
typical patients)?

- Efficacy of care–what is the level of benefit (under ideal
circumstances)?

- Efficiency of care–what is the highest quality of care
available in the shortest time with minimum expense
and positive outcome?

- Respect and caring–how well are patients treated?
(What is the level of patient satisfaction; how well are
complaints handled?)

- Safety in the care environment–includes competency,
equipment, and standard precautions.

- Timeliness of care–is care delivered in a reasonable
time (including waiting period)?

- Cost of care–is cost reasonable to marketplace?

- Availability of care–can the patient's needs be met?

KNOWLEDGE POINT 4.6:

Sentinel Event

- An event significant enough to trigger review each time it occurs; reportable to JCAHO (e.g., patient death, rape).

Program Standards/ Mammography Criteria

MULTIPLE-CHOICE QUESTIONS

1. The rate of spontaneous nuclear transformation of a radioactive nuclide describes:
   - ____ a. exposure
   - ____ b. absorbed dose
   - ____ c. becquerel
   - ____ d. activity

2. Sources of background radiation include:
   I. airplane flights
   II. the earth
   III. body tissues
   - ____ a. I and II only
   - ____ b. I and III only
   - ____ c. II and III only
   - ____ d. I, II, and III

3. What is the average bone marrow dose for an upper GI?
   - ____ a. 1–2 mGy (100–200 mrad)
   - ____ b. 4–5 mGy (400–500 mrad)
   - ____ c. 8–10 mGy (800–1000 mrad)
   - ____ d. 20–30 mGy (2000–3000 mrad)

4. Which of the following represents the reduction of radioactive atoms in a radioactive nuclide achieved after ten half-lives?
   ____ a. 10%
   ____ b. 1%
   ____ c. 0.1%
   ____ d. 0.01%

5. Which of the following types of radiation is most easily absorbed?
   ____ a. alpha
   ____ b. beta
   ____ c. x-ray
   ____ d. gamma

6. How often must sealed sources typically be leak-tested?
   ____ a. weekly
   ____ b. quarterly
   ____ c. every six months
   ____ d. yearly

7. A linear accelerator produces:
   I.   high energy x-rays
   II. high energy electron beams
   III. high energy gamma radiation

   ____ a. I and II only
   ____ b. I and III only
   ____ c. II and III only
   ____ d. I, II, and III

8. The fundamental principles of time, distance, and shielding should be understood by all hospital personnel that might be exposed to radiation.
   ____ a. true
   ____ b. false

9. High atomic-number shielding is effective for:
   ____ a. diagnostic x-ray
   ____ b. high energy gamma
   ____ c. beta radiation
   ____ d. all of the above

10. When a state inspector comes to inspect West City Outpatient Center's Radiographic Room, he finds that the exposure for an AP abdomen (as well as other exams) has increased to the point where West City is no longer in compliance with state guidelines. The technologist exclaims, "I don't know how this could happen. We phototime all of our exposures, which guarantees consistency, doesn't it?"

    What is the most likely cause of this problem?

    ____ a. The state inspector's devices must be malfunctioning.

    ____ b. A bad batch of film is being used.

    ____ c. One or more mA stations is malfunctioning.

    ____ d. The kVp has drifted.

11. Which of the following best determines focal spot size?

    ____ a. slit camera   ____ c. star test pattern

    ____ b. pinhole camera   ____ d. wire mesh test

12. Which of the following is true?

    ____ a. The site where a personal dosimeter is worn shall be documented in radiation exposure records.

    ____ b. The RSO should be contacted for guidance on the appropriate monitor.

    ____ c. All hospital personnel shall have monitors made available to them.

    ____ d. All dosimeters shall be of a type that can measure exposures of less than 0.1 mSv (10 mrem).

13. Which of the following is (are) true?

    ____ a. Radioactive materials shall be restricted to authorized locations.

    ____ b. Warning signs shall be used for radioactive material containers.

    ____ c. Employees shall be given appropriate training and safety instructions.

    ____ d. all of the above

14. Which of the following is (are) true?
    ____ a. All radioactive materials should be stored in a secured (locked) area.
    ____ b. Food shall not be stored in the same refrigerator or freezer used for storage of radioactive materials.
    ____ c. Eating, drinking, and smoking shall be prohibited in areas where radioactive materials are stored or used.
    ____ d. all of the above

15. Which of the following is considered to be a sufficient storage period for radioactive waste?
    ____ a. one half-life
    ____ b. two half-lives
    ____ c. five half-lives
    ____ d. ten half-lives

16. Which of the following is (are) true?
    ____ a. Technologists shall be aware of the approximate amount of radiation received by their patients during each radiographic procedure used in their facility.
    ____ b. Technologists shall have access to and be familiar with state regulation regarding the safe use of radiation-producing equipment.
    ____ c. Technologists shall be informed of the approximate amount of radiation they are likely to receive for a normal workload.
    ____ d. all of the above

17. Which of the following is (are) true?
    ____ a. The maximum allowable dimensions of the x-ray beam shall never exceed the size of the image receptor for both radiographic and fluoroscopic exposures.
    ____ b. The technologist should be aware of the shielding design of the room and use equipment accordingly.

_____ c. Patients should be held only after it is determined that available restraining devices are inadequate.

_____ d. all of the above

18. Where should a personal dosimeter be worn according to the NCRP?

_____ a. at the level of the trunk when no lead apron is necessary

_____ b. at the level of the head and neck when no lead apron is necessary

_____ c. at the level of the trunk when a lead apron is necessary

_____ d. at the level of the head and neck when a lead apron is necessary

19. Which of the following is (are) true?

_____ a. Leaded aprons shall be worn during fluoroscopy, special procedures, and cardiac imaging.

_____ b. Leaded gloves shall be worn during fluoroscopy, special procedures, and cardiac imaging.

_____ c. Leaded aprons shall be worn by operators of mobile equipment.

_____ d. all of the above

20. The exposure cord shall be at least 6 feet (2m) long on mobile equipment.

_____ a. true

_____ b. false

21. Under the Safe Medical Devices Act, deaths, serious illness, and serious injury attributable to medical devices must be reported to which of the following?

_____ a. Occupational Safety and Health Administration (OSHA)

_____ b. Food and Drug Administration (FDA)

_____ c. Nuclear Regulatory Commission (NRC)

_____ d. Joint Commission on Accreditation of Healthcare Organizations (JCAHO)

22. Which form is used for making voluntary reports under the Safe Medical Devices Act?
    _____ a. 3500
    _____ b. 3500A
    _____ c. 3500B
    _____ d. 3500C

23. Which of the following are components of the Safe Medical Devices Act?
    I. adverse event reporting
    II. patient follow-up
    III. medical device tracking
    _____ a. I and II only
    _____ b. I and III only
    _____ c. II and III only
    _____ d. I, II, and III

24. Which of the following would be considered user facilities under the Safe Medical Devices Act?
    _____ a. hospitals
    _____ b. nursing homes
    _____ c. outpatient treatment centers
    _____ d. all of the above

25. Which of the following is true regarding the storage of photographic materials?
    _____ a. Store at a temperature of 60–70°F.
    _____ b. Store at a humidity ranging from 40–60%.
    _____ c. Store standing on edge.
    _____ d. all of the above

26. Why should smoking be prohibited in photographic darkrooms?
    _____ a. Ashes can produce artifacts in cassettes.
    _____ b. Smoke residue can be deposited on screens and processor detectors.
    _____ c. Smoking produces light that can fog films.
    _____ d. all of the above

27. What color should darkroom walls be painted?
    _____ a. white or light colors
    _____ b. fluorescent colors

_____ c. dark colors

_____ d. any color

28. Which of the following is a potential result of high temperature/high humidity on film?

_____ a. difficult film transport

_____ b. swelling of the screen

_____ c. perspiration resulting in increased finger marks on radiographs

_____ d. white blotches on the radiograph

29. Which of the following is true regarding the film used for testing for darkroom fog?

_____ a. It is the fastest type normally used.

_____ b. It is a film of medium speed.

_____ c. It is the slowest speed normally used.

_____ d. none of the above

30. Where does fog tend to reduce film contrast?

_____ a. low-density regions

_____ b. mid-density regions

_____ c. high-density regions

_____ d. all of the above

31. An exposure of test film in the darkroom for less than one minute should produce an increase of ___ in the ___ of the film.

_____ a. less than 0.05; low-density region

_____ b. less than 0.05; mid-density region

_____ c. more than 0.05; low-density region

_____ d. more than 0.05; mid-density region

32. Which of the following represents the sensitivity to the effects of darkroom fogging by unexposed film as compared to exposed film?

_____ a. more sensitive

_____ b. less sensitive

_____ c. just as sensitive

_____ d. none of the above

33. Which of the following is the minimum number of 14- x 17-inch films that need to be processed each day to maintain the chemicals at the appropriate activity level?
    ____ a. 15 to 25
    ____ b. 25 to 35
    ____ c. 15 to 40
    ____ d. 25 to 50

34. Which of the following methods of processor monitoring do not have demonstrated value?
    I. sensitometry
    II. bromide concentration
    III. pH
    ____ a. I and II only
    ____ b. I and III only
    ____ c. II and III only
    ____ d. I, II, and III

35. The limits (in density) for the upper control limit (UCL) and lower control limit (LCL) for speed point and average gradient on the processor control chart should be set at ±:
    ____ a. 0.05
    ____ b. 0.10
    ____ c. 0.15
    ____ d. 0.20

36. What is the correct procedure following cleaning of cross-over rollers at the end of the day?
    ____ a. They should be left out until the next day.
    ____ b. They should be left out for one hour.
    ____ c. They should be left out for five minutes.
    ____ d. They should be immediately replaced.

37. For archival purposes, staining of films should be prevented for at least ___ years; preferably for ___ years.
    ____ a. 5; 10 to 15
    ____ b. 10; 10 to 15
    ____ c. 5; 20 to 30
    ____ d. 10; 20 to 25

38. Which of the following is a useful tool in addition to fixer retention testing to ensure adequate washing of film?

_____ a. pH measurement
_____ b. bromide retention
_____ c. flow meter on the water line
_____ d. temperature gauge on the water line

39. How often should flood replenishment replace all of the developer in the tank?

_____ a. in an 8-hour workday
_____ b. in a 24-hour day
_____ c. every 16 working hours
_____ d. every 24 working hours

40. Copy films are ___ films able to reproduce densities faithfully from originals up to densities of ___.

_____ a. single-emulsion; 2.3–2.5
_____ b. single-emulsion; 3.0–3.2
_____ c. double-emulsion; 2.3–2.5
_____ d. double-emulsion; 3.0–3.2

41. For the typical diagnostic x-ray unit, it is acceptable to measure HVL at a single kVp such as 80 kVp.

_____ a. true
_____ b. false

42. One of the most valuable quality control tests for regular monitoring is measurement of the focal spot size.

_____ a. true
_____ b. false

43. How often should cables and counterweights on overhead x-ray tube systems be inspected?

_____ a. daily
_____ b. weekly
_____ c. monthly
_____ d. annually

44. Which of the following are types of tube rating charts?
I. single exposure rating charts
II. anode thermal characteristic and fluoroscopic rating charts
III. housing cooling charts

_____ a. I and II only
_____ b. I and III only
_____ c. II and III only
_____ d. I, II, and III

45. kVp can be measured with devices such as the modified Ardran and Crooks cassette or Wisconsin Test cassette within ± ___ kVp.

_____ a. 0.5
_____ b. 1
_____ c. 2
_____ d. 3

46. The fact that noninvasive measurements vary from invasive measurements by 2–5 kVp is problematic from the standpoint of quality control.

_____ a. true
_____ b. false

47. For three-phase units, to what percent should exposure times in excess of the minimum exposure time be accurate?

_____ a. 2
_____ b. 5
_____ c. 7
_____ d. 10

48. What is the acceptance limit for variance of C/kg^{-1} (mR/mAs)?
I. not more than ±10% between rooms using the same types of generators, tubes, and tables
II. not more than ±10% for a single unit over time
III. not more than ±10% at different levels of kVp.

_____ a. I and II only
_____ b. I and III only
_____ c. II and III only
_____ d. I, II, and III

49. How often should grid cassettes and stationary grids designed to clip onto a cassette be checked?

____ a. each month
_ _ b. every three months
____ c. every six months
____ d. each year

50. What is the acceptance limit for the densities of films from similar cassettes and screens exposed under similar conditions?

____ a. ±2%
____ b. ±3%
____ c. ±5%
____ d. ±10%

51. Which of the following is considered to be the final test performed after all other quality control tests?

____ a. processor sensitometry
____ b. grid alignment
____ c. phantom film evaluation
____ d. screen-film contact

52. The density of patient-equivalent phantom films produced by different units should be ± ___% of all films, and should be ± ___% of he average exposure for identical rooms.

____ a. 5, 5
____ b. 10, 15
____ c. 15, 10
____ d. 10, 10

53. On the material safety data sheets (MSDSs), what level hazard is indicated by a 1?

____ a. slight
____ b. moderate
____ c. serious
____ d. severe

54. On the material safety data sheets (MSDSs), what level hazard is indicated by a 3?
    ____ a. slight
    ____ b. moderate
    ____ c. serious
    ____ d. severe

55. CFR 1910.1030 (Occupational exposure to blood-borne pathogens) indicates that protective equipment must always be supplied to all employees.
    ____ a. true
    ____ b. false

56. Contaminated glassware can be picked up with the hands as long as the employee wears durable gloves.
    ____ a. true
    ____ b. false

57. An employer must make the hepatitis B vaccine "available" to employees with occupational exposure, but the employee must pay for it.
    ____ a. true
    ____ b. false

58. Which of the following is true regarding the hepatitis B vaccine provided to all employees?
    ____ a. The vaccine must be provided before they begin their work assignment.
    ____ b. The vaccine must be provided the day they begin their work assignment.
    ____ c. The vaccine must be provided within a week of work assignment.
    ____ d. The vaccine must be provided within 10 days of work assignment.

59. Employees cannot refuse a hepatitis B vaccine.
    ____ a. true
    ____ b. false

60. It is necessary to secure an employee's consent to have blood drawn post-exposure to potential HBV/HIV.

_____ a. true

_____ b. false

61. If an employee consents to baseline blood collection, but does not give consent for HIV serologic testing, how long must the sample be preserved?

_____ a. 30 days

_____ b. 60 days

_____ c. 90 days

_____ d. indefinitely

62. Red bags or red containers may be substituted for warning labels for infectious materials.

_____ a. true

_____ b. false

63. Regulated waste that has been decontaminated need not be labeled or color-coded.

_____ a. true

_____ b. false

64. When must training for employees with potential occupational exposure be conducted?

I. at the time of initial assignment to tasks with potential exposure

II. whenever standards change

III. annually

_____ a. I and II only

_____ b. I and III only

_____ c. II and III only

_____ d. I, II, and III

65. How long must medical records for employee exposure be kept after the employment ends?

_____ a. 5

_____ b. 10

_____ c. 20

_____ d. 30

66. How long must training records be maintained?
    ____ a. 1 year
    ____ b. 3 years
    ____ c. 5 years
    ____ d. 10 years

67. Employees cannot engage in work activities involving infectious agents until proficiency has been demonstrated?
    ____ a. true
    ____ b. false

68. If an employee refuses the initial HBV vaccination, a later vaccination must be provided if the employee desires, but the employee must bear the cost of the vaccination series.
    ____ a. true
    ____ b. false

69. Which of the following describes controls such as Sharps disposal containers that isolate or remove a bloodborne pathogens hazard from the workplace?
    ____ a. workplace controls
    ____ b. exposure controls
    ____ c. occupational controls
    ____ d. engineering controls

70. Which of the following should be used to make an employee aware of unsafe chemicals in the work environment?
    ____ a. Physicians Desk Reference (PDR)
    ____ b. Periodic Table
    ____ c. Material Safety Data Sheet (MSDS)
    ____ d. Code of Federal Regulations (CFR)

71. For mammography phantom radiography, the minimum number of objects required to pass ACR accreditation is ___ fibers, ___ speck groups, and ___ masses.
    ____ a. 2, 3, 4
    ____ b. 3, 3, 3
    ____ c. 4, 3, 3
    ____ d 4, 4, 4

72. In phantom radiography for ACR mammography accreditation, if half of the fiber is shown and in the correct location and orientation, a score of 0.5 is given.

_____ a. true
_____ b. false

73. In phantom radiography for ACR mammography accreditation, if two or more of the speck group are visible, a full point is given.

_____ a. true
_____ b. false

74. In phantom radiography for ACR mammography accreditation if the shape of the mass is not circular, the score is zero.

_____ a. true
_____ b. false

75. At 80 kVp, changes of 2 or 3 kVp will typically change HVL by ___ mm Al eq.

_____ a. 0.1
_____ b. 0.5
_____ c. 1.0
_____ d. 1.5

76. Where should the device be placed when performing quality assurance tests that take measurements from film, such as the kVp test cassette, or a step wedge?

_____ a. perpendicular to the anode-cathode axis
_____ b. parallel with the anode-cathode axis
_____ c. toward the cathode end of the tube
_____ d. toward the anode end of the tube

77. Which of the following chemicals would require wearing gloves and goggles when mixing a developer solution?

_____ a. sodium carbonate
_____ b. sodium sulfite
_____ c. sodium hydroxide
_____ d. all of the above

ANSWERS TO CHAPTER 2 PROGRAM STANDARDS/MAMMOGRAPHY CRITERIA QUESTIONS

1. **d**   Exposure is a measure of ionization caused by the absorption of x-rays in a specified mass of air at the point of interest; absorbed dose is the amount of radiation absorbed in matter; becquerel is one of the units (along with curie) used to specify exposure; and activity is the rate of spontaneous nuclear transformation of a radioactive nuclide.

2. **d**   Sources of radiation include the earth and sky, and increased altitudes increase one's radiation exposure. Body tissues themselves contain radioactive atoms, including potassium-40.

3. **b**   Both an upper GI and a lumbar spine series will provide about 4–5 mGy of bone marrow exposure.

4. **c**   During each half-life, 50% of the atoms will be transformed; thus 10 half-lives, less than 1/10 of 1% (0.1%) of the radioactive atoms will remain.

5. **a**   Alpha emitters are rarely used in medicine, and are easily absorbed in air; beta particles can penetrate a few mm into living tissue; and gamma and x-rays have a wide range of penetrating ability, dependent on energy.

6. **c**   Unless specifically exempted, sealed sources used for teletherapy and brachytherapy must be leak-tested at least every six months to ensure detection of inadvertent escape of the radioactive material.

7. **a**   When energized, linear accelerators produce high-energy x-rays. They can also produce high-energy electron beams useful for shallow depth tumors, such as those of the skin or head and neck.

8. **a**   The protection factors of time, distance, and shielding should be understood by all hospital personnel who might be potentially exposed due to wide uses of radiation throughout the hospital. Note however, that

occasional exposure in the course of one's job duties does not necessarily make one an "occupationally exposed worker."

9. **a** Lead shielding is most valuable for diagnostic x-rays; plexiglass shielding is often used for beta because beta particles convert their energy to x-ray upon interaction with matter; and lead shielding may not be effective for high-energy gamma radiation.

10. **d** It is most likely that the kVp has drifted downward, and the automatic exposure device (phototimer) has compensated for this by increasing mAs, which has increased patient exposure to unacceptable levels. One clue might be a change in the contrast of images; however, since lower kV most likely improved the contrast scale, it may have gone unnoticed.

11. **a** The slit camera, according to the NEMA standards, is the best method used to determine focal spot size, modulation transfer function, and focal spot blooming. Orientation and intensity distribution are best determined with the pinhole camera. The Star test pattern is used to measure limits of resolution.

12. **b** The site where a personal dosimeter is worn should be documented in radiation exposure records; the RSO should be contacted for guidance on the appropriate monitor; monitoring is not essential for all personnel, and most dosimeters used to monitor personnel cannot accurately record exposures of less than 0.1–0.2 mSv (10–20 mrem) and represent these as "M" or minimal.

13. **d** Radioactive materials should be restricted to authorized locations; warning signs should be used for radioactive material containers; and employees should be given appropriate training and safety instructions.

14. **d** All radioactive materials should be stored in a secured (locked) area; food should not be stored in the same refrigerator or freezer used for storage of radioactive materials; and eating, drinking, and smoking shall be prohibited in areas where radioactive materials are stored or used.

15. **d**   Following ten half-lives, and surveying the material with the right instruments, materials can be considered non-radioactive. Other means of managing waste, in addition to storage for decay, include shipment for burial, release to the environment, and release to the sanitary sewer.

16. **d**   Technologists shall be aware of the approximate amount of radiation received by their patients during each radiographic procedure used in their facility; should have access to and be familiar with state regulations regarding the safe use of radiation-producing equipment; and should be informed of the approximate amount of radiation they are likely to receive for a normal workload within their assigned working area.

17. **d**   The maximum allowance dimensions of the x-ray beam shall never exceed the size of the image receptor for both radiographic and fluoroscopic exposures; the technologist should be aware of the shielding design of the room and use equipment accordingly; patients should be held only after it is determined that available restraining devices are inadequate.

18. **a**   A variety of potential uses of the dosimeter with and without an apron are described in NCRP #105; the one firm recommendation is that the dosimeter should be worn at trunk level when no lead apron is necessary. This recommendation may conflict with other recommendations.

19. **a**   Leaded aprons should be worn during fluoroscopy, special procedures, and cardiac imaging; lead gloves should be worn during fluoroscopy, special procedures, and cardiac imaging; and leaded aprons should be worn by operators of mobile equipment.

20. **b**   The cord to the exposure switch for mobile equipment should be long enough to permit the operator to be at least 2m (6 feet) from the patient during an exposure; this does not mean that the cord must be 2m (6 feet). In fact, if the console of the machine is large enough to permit the operator to be adequately shielded by the console, the exposure cord should be short to encourage the operator to remain behind the console.

21. b   The Safe Medical Devices Act of 1990 requires that both manufacturers and user facilities report to the Food and Drug Administration (FDA) deaths, serious injury, and illness attributed to medical devices.

22. a   The MedWatch reporting program was implemented in June 1993 by the FDA, providing two forms: Form 3500, for voluntary reporting, and Form 3500A for mandatory reporting.

23. b   The two major components of SMDA are adverse event reporting and medical device tracking. Medical device tracking went into effect in August of 1993.

24. d   SMDA defines hospitals, nursing homes, outpatient treatment centers, and ambulatory surgical facilities as user facilities. Physician offices and group practices that implant or distribute tracked devices are also regulated under the tracking rule.

25. d   In addition to being a photosensitive material, photographic film is also sensitive to heat, humidity, chemicals, mechanical stress, and ambient radiation. These materials should be stored at temperatures less than 24°C (75°F), with a range of 15–21°C (60–70°F) preferred. Once film is opened it should be stored in an area with humidity ranging between 40–60%.

26. d   Eating, drinking, and smoking should not be allowed in any darkroom. Smoking can produce artifacts in cassettes, smoke residue can be deposited on screens and processor detectors, and smoking in the darkroom would produce light that can fog film.

27. a   White or light colors are preferred, as it will help vision when illumination levels are low. Counter tops should also be white or a light color.

28. c   Humidity above 60% may make films sticky and difficult to handle, while high temperature and/or high humidity can cause perspiration resulting in finger marks. Either high or low humidity can cause difficult film transport.

29.   **a**   The fastest film normally used in the darkroom should be used for the darkroom fog test, and if more than one type of film is used, the fastest film of each type should be tested.

30.   **b**   Film fogging reduces film contrast in the regions of the film most important to producing a quality image, the mid-density regions of the film.

31.   **b**   There should be an increase of less than 0.05 in fog in the mid-density region of the film (density of about 1.20), and ideally less than an 0.05 increase should be seen at this region with the two-minute exposure to the safelight.

32.   **b**   Unexposed films are less sensitive to darkroom fogging than exposed films due to a threshold effect.

33.   **d**   Most mechanized processors require a minimum of 25–50 14- x 17-inch films be processed each day to maintain chemical activity in the processor. If this is not possible, various adjustments can be made, such as flood replenishment or changes in the replenishment rate (if volume is sufficient, but mostly small films are being processed, as in mammography).

34.   **c**   Due to the complexity of chemical interactions in the solution and the many chemicals in the solution, pH and bromide concentration have not been proven to be of value in processor monitoring.

35.   **b**   The upper control limit (UCL) and lower control limit (LCL) for mid-density and density should be set at ± 0.10.

36.   **a**   At the end of the work day, the cross-over rollers are cleaned with warm water and a damp, soft cloth, and dried. However, these rollers are not replaced until the start of the next day.

37.   **d**   Staining is prevented by ensuring that films are stored at the proper conditions of 21°C. (70°F), and a humidity of 40–60%, in addition to adequate washing. Staining should be prevented for at least 10 years, and preferably 20 to 25 years.

38.　c　A flow meter is valuable in ensuring adequate washing, but especially when water must be filtered to ensure the removal of particulate matter before reaching the processor.

39.　c　Flood replenishment automatically adds a predetermined amount of modified replenisher at specified time intervals, and is selected so that all of the develop in the developer tanks is replaced every 16 working hours.

40.　c　Single-emulsion films are unable to reproduce all densities on a radiograph; copy films can typically reproduce the densities on an original film up to 2.3 to 2.5.

41.　a　It is acceptable to measure HVL at one kVp; HVL should be measured annually and whenever x-ray tubes are replaced or engineers service the x-ray tube or collimator. One common mistake is not replacing or adding filtration.

42.　b　Although all focal spots should be measured as a part of acceptance testing, and whenever tubes are replaced there is no value to regular monitoring of focal spot size.

43.　d　Cables and counterweights should be inspected at least annually, and should be lubricated with the assistance of a service engineer as directed by the manufacturer.

44.　d　Types of tube and housing rating charts include single exposure rating charts specific to focal spot size, anode rotation speed, and generator; anode thermal characteristic and fluoroscopic rating charts; housing cooling charts; and angiographic and cine rating charts. If an x-ray tube sensor is used, it should be set to provide a warning when anode heat reaches 75% of maximum.

45. d   The modified Ardran and Crooks cassette is accurate ±3 kVp whereas noninvasive measuring devices are accurate ± 2% with a reproducibility of ±0.5 kVp.

46. b   The accuracy of kVp need only be measured initially; thereafter, measures of consistency provided by the Ardran and Crooks cassette are sufficient from the standpoint of quality control.

47. b   For three-phase units, exposure times above the minimum exposure time should be accurate ±5%. For single-phase units, the acceptance limits are ±1 dot for 1/5 and 1/ 16 second, and ±0 dots for 1/20 and 1/30 second.

48. a   The C kg^{-1}(mR)/mAs, measured at 80 kVp, should be maintained to within ±10% among rooms using the same types of generators, tubes, and tables. If not, unless exposures are predominantly automated, different technique charts are needed. On a single unit, it should not vary more than ±10% over time. It should be measured at least annually.

49. c   Grid cassettes and stationary grids designed to clip onto a cassette should be checked at least every six months if the grid appears to be damaged, or if the grid is suspected of creating artifacts.

50. c   The light output of screen doses changes with age, and cassettes that produce film densities outside of the range of ±5% should be taken out of service or isolated.

51. c   The use of a phantom as the last quality control check ensures that proper images can be produced, helps monitor differences in exposure, and can indicate whether problems are a result of equipment or personnel problems.

52. c   The density of all patient-equivalent phantom films produced by different units should be within ±15% of all film, and entrance exposures should be within ±10% of the average exposure for identical rooms. If the difference in exposure is due to certain factors (e.g., HVL or technique), such variation should be reduced by standardizing these parameters.

53. **a** On the MSDS, 1 would be slight hazard, 2 moderate, 3 serious, and 4 severe.

54. **c** On the MSDS, 1 would be a slight hazard, 2 moderate, 3 serious, and 4 severe.

55. **b** CFR 1910.1030 (Occupational exposure to bloodborne pathogens) indicates that protective equipment must always be supplied to all employees.

56. **b** Broken or contaminated glassware cannot be picked up with the hands according to CFR 910.1030 (Occupational exposure to bloodborne pathogens), but shall be cleaned up using mechanical means such as brush and dust pan, tongs, or forceps.

57. **b** According to CFR 910.1030 (Occupational exposure to bloodborne pathogens), the employer must make the vaccine available to the employee at no cost, as well as available at a reasonable time and place, and performed by an appropriately licensed health professional.

58. **d** According to CFR 910.1030, the hepatitis B vaccine must be provided to all employees within 10 days of work assignment unless the vaccination is contraindicated for medical reasons, the employee is immune (as shown through antibody testing), or the vaccine has been previously received.

59. **b** Employees can refuse the hepatitis B vaccine.

60. **a** For post-exposure to HBV/HIV, the exposed employee's blood should be collected as soon as feasible, after consent has been received. The employee may also consent to have only baseline blood collection done and if he or she consents within 90 days to have HIV testing performed, it shall be done as soon as feasible.

61. **c** If an employee consents to baseline blood collection, but does not give consent for HIV serologic testing, the sample shall be preserved for at least 90 days. The employee may also consent to have only baseline blood collection done, and if he or she consents within

90 days to have HIV testing performed, it shall be done as soon as feasible.

62. a Although the orange or orange-red label typically indicates a biohazard is used, it is acceptable to substitute red bags or red containers for labels.

63. a Once regulated waste has been decontaminated, it is no longer required to label or color-code it.

64. d Training program records for employees with occupational exposure must be provided at the time of initial assignment, within 90 days after the effective date of the standard, at least annually thereafter, and whenever standards change.

65. d Medical records to include hepatitis B vaccination status must be maintained for at least the duration of employment plus 30 years.

66. b Training program records must be maintained for at least 3 years, and must contain the dates of the training session, the contents or summary of the session, the names and qualifications of those providing the training, and the names and job titles of all attending the session.

67. a The training program and the assignment of work duties must follow a logical progression, and employees cannot engage in work activities involving infectious material until they are proficient to do so.

68. b The cost of the vaccination is always bore by the employer.

69. d Controls such as Sharps disposal containers that isolate or remove a bloodborne pathogens hazard from the workplace are known as engineering controls.

70. c Employees are made aware of unsafe chemicals in the work environment through the MSDS or Material Safety Data Sheet.

71. c For radiography of the mammography phantom the minimum number of objects required to pass ACR accreditation is 4 fibers, 3 speck groups, and 3 masses.

72. a   In phantom radiography by ACR mammography accreditation, if half of the fiber is shown and in the correct location orientation, a score of 0.5 is given. The score is 1 applies if the entire fiber is visible at the correct location and orientation, and zero if less than half is visible.

73. b   In phantom radiography by ACR mammography accreditation, if four or more of the six specks are visible a full point is given. The score of 0.5 is given if two are visible, and zero if less than two are visible.

74. b   In phantom radiography for ACR mammography accreditation, if the shape of the mass is not circular, but the density difference is at the correct location, the score is 0.5. It is given a full point if the density difference is seen at the correct location with a circular border, and zero if there is only a hint of a density difference seen.

75. a   Change of 2 or 3 kVp at about 80 kVp will change HVL by about 0.1 mm Al eq.

76. a   The heel effect is the change in intensity of the x-ray beam along the anode-cathode axis. Placing devices perpendicular to the axis will ensure a minimal variation in intensity along the length of the device.

77. c   Sodium hydroxide is the strongest alkali, commonly called lye. It is very corrosive and can eat away at the skin, requiring gloves and goggles.

Quality Improvement Concepts

MULTIPLE-CHOICE QUESTIONS

1. Which of the following is (are) true regarding Deming's 14 points?
    ____ a. It has specific managerial structure.
    ____ b. Its emphasis is on management by objectives.
    ____ c. It has process orientation.
    ____ d. all of the above

2. Which of the following are philosophical foundations of CQI?
    I.   Systems View
    II. Implementer Involvement
    III. Single Causation
    ____ a. I and II only
    ____ b. I and III only
    ____ c. II and III only
    ____ d. I, II, and III

3. The primary decision-making criteria for CQI is price.
    ____ a. true
    ____ b. false

4. Which of the following would be considered internal customers in a hospital?
    I.   physicians
    II. employees
    III. patients

    ____ a. I and II only
    ____ b. I and III only
    ____ c. II and III only
    ____ d. I, II, and III

5. Which of the following are considered customers in a CQI system?
    I.   patient
    II. provider
    III. payer

    ____ a. I and II only
    ____ b. I and III only
    ____ c. II and III only
    ____ d. I, II, and III

6. Most participants in CQI can be considered both customers and suppliers.
    ____ a. true
    ____ b. false

7. Which of the following is the best source for information about quality?
    ____ a. supplier
    ____ b. customer
    ____ c. employee
    ____ d. manager

8. What is the function of management in CQI, according to Deming?
    ____ a. Be responsible for data collection.
    ____ b. Provide rewards and punishment for performance.
    ____ c. Track down the causes of poor performance.
    ____ d. Optimize the system.

9. What is the main reason for failure of a team?
   ____ a. unskilled leadership
   ____ b. lack of effective training
   ____ c. unclear goals, including lack of adequate customer definition
   ____ d. dysfunctional behavior by team members

10. Which of the following is (are) phase(s) in the formation and use of CQI teams?
    ____ a. orientation
    ____ b. development
    ____ c. reiteration
    ____ d. all of the above

11. Which of the following would be useful in documenting problems with patient transport?
    I.   flowchart
    II. cause-effect diagram
    III. Pareto chart

    ____ a. I and II only
    ____ b. I and III only
    ____ c. II and III only
    ____ d. I, II, and III

12. Which of the following is expressed by the statement, "Whenever a quality problem has multiple causes, just a few of those causes account for most of the incidents"?
    ____ a. Deming's first principle
    ____ b. crosstab incidence
    ____ c. the Pareto principle
    ____ d. the quality improvement principle

13. It is not necessary to investigate the cause if a control chart is consistently on the low end (more than eight occurrences) as long as it does not exceed control limits.
    ____ a. true
    ____ b. false

14. How many standard deviations represent the limits of a control chart for CQI?
    ___ a. one
    ___ b. two
    ___ c. three
    ___ d. four

15. What term describes a chart that documents the mean?
    ___ a. x-bar chart
    ___ b. s-bar chart
    ___ c. r-bar chart
    ___ d. p-chart

16. Which of the following is frequently used late in the quality improvement process to answer the question, "Are we doing better?"
    ___ a. run chart
    ___ b. control chart
    ___ c. cause-and-effect diagram
    ___ d. histogram

17. Which of the following describes a bar chart that does not provide the ordering of a Pareto chart?
    ___ a. run chart
    ___ b. control chart
    ___ c. cause-and-effect diagram
    ___ d. histogram

18. Which of the following is (are) consistent with a focus on continuity of care?
    ___ a. The same level of care is provided throughout the care setting.
    ___ b. If nurses give injections on the floor, nurses should also be responsible for giving injections in radiology.
    ___ c. Floor nurses should accompany their patients throughout the hospital.
    ___ d. all of the above

19. If level 1 is the lowest level of understanding the needs of customers, and level 3 is the highest, which of the following is (are) most likely to bring about a level 3 understanding?

    ____ a. unsolicited complaints
    ____ b. telephone hotline
    ____ c. focus groups
    ____ d. all of the above

20. Which of the following describes the potential effect of the time of day a survey is given on customer response?

    ____ a. environmental contaminant
    ____ b. reliability variation
    ____ c. validity deficit
    ____ d. response-set bias

21. Which of the following indicates reproducibility of measures on a survey?

    ____ a. reliability
    ____ b. construct validity
    ____ c. content validity
    ____ d. criterion validity

22. Which of the following is the greatest reliability in a measure of central tendency?

    ____ a. mean
    ____ b. median
    ____ c. mode
    ____ d. standard deviation

23. Which of the following is appropriate if one is interested in whether cases fall only within upper and lower halves of the distribution and not how far from the central point?

    ____ a. mean
    ____ b. median
    ____ c. mode
    ____ d. standard deviation

24. What is calculated if one wants to determine the most typical case?
   ____ a. mean
   ____ b. median
   ____ c. mode
   ____ d. standard deviation

25. What is calculated if interpretations about the normal distribution curve are needed?
   ____ a. mean
   ____ b. median
   ____ c. mode
   ____ d. standard deviation

26. What tests one or more hypotheses indicating that the means of all groups sampled come from populations with equal means, differing only because of sampling error?
   ____ a. standard deviation
   ____ b. range
   ____ c. simple correlation
   ____ d. analysis of variance

27. Range/6 is approximately equal to how many standard deviation(s) when the sample size is approximately 100?
   ____ a. one   ____ c. four
   ____ b. two   ____ d. six

28. An analysis of contrast reactions for the past year shows 20 reactions that were serious, and 15 of those came from patients above the age of 65. Which of the following is a reasonable conclusion?
   ____ a. Younger patients are not as prone to contrast reactions.
   ____ b. There were more serious reactions in the older population.
   ____ c. Older patients should be considered primary candidates for non-ionic contrast.
   ____ d. All of the above are reasonable conclusions.

29. Which of the following process measures (professional performance) is (are) of most use?
    ____ a. when an accepted standard of care exists
    ____ b. when technology is effective
    ____ c. when patient variables (level of illness, age, etc.) are controlled
    ____ d. all of the above

30. The assumption that a hospital with a lower rate of adverse consequences is producing the better patient outcomes is reasonable.
    ____ a. true
    ____ b. false

31. What terms describes adjusting for differences in case mix and case complexity?
    ____ a. outcomes analysis
    ____ b. epidemiology
    ____ c. risk adjustment
    ____ d. risk management

32. Which of the following first established corporate liability of hospitals?
    ____ a. HCFA mortality data
    ____ b. HMOs
    ____ c. PPOs
    ____ d. The *Darling v. Charleston Memorial Hospital* case

33. Which of the following is (are) the goal(s) of benchmarking?
    ____ a. identify best practices in related settings
    ____ b. identify best practices in unrelated settings
    ____ c. find ways to emulate best practices or use them as performance standards
    ____ d. all of the above

34. What term describes standards that reflect the best practices of medicine?

_____ a. institutional

_____ b. empirical

_____ c. absolute (normative)

_____ d. internal

35. Both poor and good handling of data can make a hospital's outcomes look worse.

_____ a. true

_____ b. false

36. Which of the following is the most direct customer of a requisition for a chest x-ray generated by the admissions desk of a hospital?

_____ a. patient

_____ b. staff technologist

_____ c. chief technologist

_____ d. physician

37. Which term related to qualify is most synonymous with quality assurance?

_____ a. conformance quality

_____ b. quality of kind

_____ c. requirements quality

_____ d. total quality

38. IN CQI, the causes of a problem are determined based on which of the following?

_____ a. institution

_____ b. customer opinion

_____ c. empirical data

_____ d. management's decision

39. Which of the following is the most appropriate statement of a quality goal?

_____ a. Quality is our most important product.

_____ b. This year we will work to improve our customers' satisfaction.

_____ c. No one will leave our department dissatisfied.

_____ d. During this quarter, we will reduce patient waiting time to no more than 10 minutes after arrival in the department.

40. The expression "quality is free" means that it costs nothing additional to implement a CQI plan.

    ____ a. true

    ____ b. false

41. Crosby was a proponent of which of the following ideas?

    ____ a. "Zero defects" is the only performance standard.

    ____ b. The costs of quality are less than the losses of nonquality.

    ____ c. Conform to requirements to perform a task correctly on the first try.

    ____ d. all of the above

42. CQI techniques are applied only to processes where problems have been identified.

    ____ a. true

    ____ b. false

43. Approximately how long does it take for an organization to transform itself by implementing CQI techniques?

    ____ a. 6 months

    ____ b. 1 year

    ____ c. 5 years

    ____ d. 10 years

44. In health care organizations, medical specialization adversely affects which of the following essential components of CQI?

    ____ a. knowledge

    ____ b. commitment

    ____ c. communication

    ____ d. patience

45. One of the benefits that results from a CQI program is increased employee satisfaction with the work environment.

    ____ a. true

    ____ b. false

46. The cost of waste and nonconformance in the health
care system has been estimated to be what percentage of total costs associated with health care?
_____ a. less than 10%
_____ b. 20% to 40%
_____ c. 55% to 60%
_____ d. over 75%

47. While multidisciplinary teams are generally
regarded as desirable in CQI, their diversity may
also interfere with their functioning.
_____ a. true
_____ b. false

48. Which of the following describes a process owner
who is a member of a CQI team?
I.   supports the improvement process
II. hinders the improvement process
III. holds an upper level administrative position

_____ a. I and II only
_____ b. I and III only
_____ c. II and III only
_____ d. I, II, and III

49. A successful team experiences high level of both situational conflict and interpersonal conflict.
_____ a. true
_____ b. false

50. All of the following characteristics are consistent
with the CQI/TQM philosophy *except*:
_____ a. collective responsibilities
_____ b. accountability
_____ c. professional autonomy
_____ d. process expectations

51. The concept of benchmarking includes which of the
following actions?
_____ a. responding only as problems arise
_____ b. changing based on the values of services
providers

_____ c. doing things the same way for a long time

_____ d. comparing products and processes to those of the best competitor

52. On of the chief functions of top management in a CQI organization is to distribute resources to support the changes in processes.

_____ a. true

_____ b. false

53. Why is it especially important for academic health centers to become involved in CQI?

_____ a. They set the standards for patient care

_____ b. They educate most of the physicians in the United States

_____ c. They conduct a significant portion of research that affects health care

_____ d. all of the above

54. Which of the following is the most significant conflict between management and practitioners in the health care setting?

_____ a. the quality of clinical care

_____ b. relationships with patients

_____ c. cost reduction

_____ d. professional reputations

55. Which of the following is the best measure of team performance?

_____ a. quality of work products

_____ b. amount of time needed to solve the problem

_____ c. leader performance

_____ d. developing a large number of work products

56. Which of the following typically describes CQI teams?

_____ a. They are ineffective.

_____ b. They outperform individuals acting alone.

_____ c. They provide minimal opportunity for advancement.

_____ d. They are not cost-effective.

57. How does management influence team effectiveness?

_____ a. by being directive

_____ b. by demanding rapid solutions

_____ c. by demonstrating the significance of effort

_____ d. by providing the team's work rules

58. Who provided the earliest known method of evaluating quality of clinical care by assessing patient outcomes?

_____ a. Deming _____ c. Codman

_____ b. Donabedian _____ d. Nightingale

59. Which of the following is (are) component(s) of a good team?

_____ a. a small number of individuals

_____ b. individuals with complimentary skills

_____ c. individuals with a common purpose

_____ d. all of the above

60. Which of the following is (are) related to the statement: "Cooperating departments with the best intentions often lose sight of subtle slippage in effectiveness and efficiency"?

_____ a. Slippage is seen as an acceptable post-implementation adjustment.

_____ b. Slippage can be reduced by a dedicated individual in the institution monitoring CQI efforts.

_____ c. Periodic meetings with employees (team members) and mangers are useful.

_____ d. all of the above

61. Which of the following best accomplishes reducing average length of stay?

I. long-term purchase contracts

II. developing critical pathways

III. improving discharging planning

_____ a. I and II only

_____ b. I and III only

_____ c. II and III only

_____ d. I, II, and III

62. Which of the following are elements of a well-developed CQI program?

I.   identify all customers for each service

II. development of a CQI panel

III. strong, directive management policies

____   a. I and II only

____   b. I and III only

____   c. II and III only

____   d. I, II, and III

63. How does CQI define "process"?

____   a. the steps required to provide care

____   b. a series of steps that achieve a desired outcome

____   c. patient care activities

____   d. technical aspects of providing care

64. Which of the following is (are) most likely to describe how CQI can save money?

____   a. reduce time spent on training

____   b. reduce time spent on meetings

____   c. reduce labor and material waste

____   d. all of the above

65. A sentinel event is a single negative outcome focused on by a CQI team.

____   a. true

____   b. false

66. What are the four foundational elements of the quality improvement process as seen in the Shewhart cycle?

____   a. find, organize, clarify, understand

____   b. plan, do, check, act

____   c. find, plan, organize, do

____   d. plan, find, check, act

67. Which of the following represents an activity in a flowchart?

____   a. rectangle

____   b. oval

____   c. triangle

____   d. quadrangle

68. Which of the following are ranking mechanisms used in group decision-making?

    ____ a. multivoting

    ____ b. rank ordering

    ____ c. both of the above

    ____ d. none of the above

69. How would a CQI team most likely view the development of a new method of ordering "stat" examinations to deal with excessive "stat" exams—superstat?

    ____ a. a good idea

    ____ b. the problem of excessive stat exams has not been dealt with

    ____ c. we should brainstorm and collect data first

    ____ d. two of the above

70. Who is the primary customer in the production of a report based on the radiologist's reading of a film?

    ____ a. radiologist

    ____ b. referring physician

    ____ c. patient

    ____ d. transcriptionist

71. Who is the primary customer when the insurance company pays a patient's bill for a barium enema?

    ____ a. insurance company

    ____ b. referring physician

    ____ c. technologist

    ____ d. hospital/radiology department

72. Which of the following are true about employees as customers?

    I. They require services from other employees to perform their job and are known as external customers.

    II. Job dissatisfaction is a factor in making them less effective in handling customers.

    III. They serve a marketing function by serving as representatives of the institution to friends, family, and acquaintances.

_____ a. I and II only
_____ b. II and III only
_____ c. I and III only
_____ d. I, II, and III

73. Third-party customers see which of the following as important?
_____ a. cost
_____ b. quality of clinical services
_____ c. ease of administration and accuracy
_____ d. all of the above

74. Which of the following is (are) true?
_____ a. It cost about 5–10 times as much to recruit a new customer than to retain an old one.
_____ b. Most customers will not continue to do business with an organization with which they have problems, regardless of attempts by that organization to solve the problem.
_____ c. Complainers are the least likely to return to an organization with which they had problems.
_____ d. all of the above

75. Which of the following is (are) imperative for the survey administered following customer service training?
_____ a. that it be criterion-based
_____ b. that it measures changes in participant's attitudes
_____ c. that it evaluates effectiveness of presentation and appropriateness of content
_____ d. all of the above

76. Which of the following has been identified as the most important aspect of customer service to physicians?
_____ a. new technology
_____ b. efficient personnel
_____ c. quick access to other physicians
_____ d. services that contribute to their ease of practice

77. What term describes the process for correcting customer complaints?
    ____ a. malpractice adjustment
    ____ b. risk management
    ____ c. service recovery
    ____ d. focus feedback

78. In which of the following scenarios in the customer-supplier chain is the patient the primary customer?
    I. patient comes to physician complaining of low back pain
    II. technologist performs lumbar spine x-ray
    II. hospital sends bill to third-party payer

    ____ a. I and II only
    ____ b. I and III only
    ____ c. II and III only
    ____ d. I, II, and III

79. For which examination might the patient be both customer and supplier?
    ____ a. lumbar spine
    ____ b. barium enema
    ____ c. mammography
    ____ d. none of the above

80. According the principle of TQM, who has the most intimate knowledge of an organization's work?
    ____ a. management
    ____ b. central administration
    ____ c. workers
    ____ d. all have different understanding of the same work

81. What advantages include employee contributions to the improving the work environment according to TQM theory?
    I. sense of ownership
    II. reduces adversarial relationships
    III. improves profitability

____   a. I and II only
____   b. I and III only
____   c. II and III only
____   d. I, II, and III

82. What is the primary difference between TQM and CQI?

____   a. a TQM is a management philosophy while CQI is a data collection and analysis technique.
____   b. TQM is a public/employee relations approach and CQI is the evaluation technique for that approach
____   c. both a and b are true
____   d. neither a nor b are true

83. Which of the following is a major difference QA and QM?

I.   standards of acceptability are set
II. quality outcomes are the goal
III. the focus of the process is the problems

____   a. I and II only
____   b. I and III only
____   c. II and III only
____   d. I, II, and III

84. Which of the following is not a component of quality Improvement (QI)?

____   a. developed locally and responds to the needs of the organization
____   b. customer and supplier satisfaction
____   c. rewards employee contributions
____   d. nurtures the professional instinct for continuous self-assessment and improvement through evaluation of variations over time

85. According to Deming's 14 points, what is the function of mass inspection of products?
    ____ a. used to develop statistical profile of quality
    ____ b. allows for prospective quality measures
    ____ c. helps keep employees honest and productive
    ____ d. such inspections are counter productive

86. What are the fundamental aspects of any job-related training program?
    I.   job responsibilities and how to accomplish them
    II. cross training where effective or useful
    III. basic statistical control methods

    ____ a. I and II only
    ____ b. I and III only
    ____ c. II and III only
    ____ d. I, II, and III

87. What are some of the possible outcomes of using a merit rating system?
    I.   pride in workmanship increases
    II. creates rivalries and destroys teams
    III. directs work toward evaluation rather than quality

    ____ a. I and II only
    ____ b. I and III only
    ____ c. II and III only
    ____ d. I, II, and III

88. In an organization, who is responsible for knowing and understanding the vision, mission, and guiding principles?
    ____ a. everyone
    ____ b. only managers
    ____ c. only manager and QM personnel
    ____ d. it doesn't matter as they have no impact of organizational action

89. Which of the following are criteria any vision statement should meet?
I.   have consistency of purpose
II. be simple and easily understood
III. be energizing, compelling, and inspiring

_____ a. I and II only   _____ c. II and III only
_____ b. I and III only   _____ d. I, II, and III

90. Which of the following are aspects of a good mission statement?
I.   clearly defines the product of the organization
II. defines the scope of individual responsibility
III. clearly defines the efficiency goals of the organization

_____ a. I and II only   _____ c. II and III only
_____ b. I and III only   _____ d. I, II, and III

91. What are the functions of guiding principles?
I.   Empower employees to carry out the aims of the organization without micromanagement.
II. Clearly define lines of authority within the organization.
III. Enhance the flavor of the organization as established in the mission and vision statements.

_____ a. I and II only
_____ b. I and III only
_____ c. II and III only
_____ d. I, II, and III

92. When designing customer satisfaction surveys, which of the following is not acceptable?
_____ a. must be administered by an employee
_____ b. must be short, precise, and concise
_____ c. should include demographic variables
_____ d. should allow for multiple responses to most questions

93. What are KQCs?

_____ a. aspects of the service important to the customer

_____ b. measurement points for quality control

_____ c. the ratio between manpower commitment and customer satisfaction

_____ d. none of the above

94. In quality management, KVPs have what characteristics?

I. contain the cause and effect of process variable

II. related to manpower, machines, material, methods, environment, and measures of the system

III. compare the cost of the product to the customer satisfaction

_____ a. I and II only

_____ b. I and III only

_____ c. II and III only

_____ d. I, II, and III only

95. Who are the customers of the radiology receptionist?

_____ a. referring physician

_____ b. patients

_____ c. technologists

_____ d. all of the above

96. Which of the following are steps in quality measurement?

I. defining the process

II. defining the KQCs

III. creating data collection plan

_____ a. I and II only

_____ b. I and III only

_____ c. II and III only

_____ d. I, II, and III

97. What is operational definition?
_____ a. a well worded definition?
_____ b. explicit directions on how something is evaluated
_____ c. a definition based on a proven theory
_____ d. any definition related to the operation of equipment

98. Which of the following is not one of the five steps in a process?
_____ a. action
_____ b. output
_____ c. evaluation
_____ d. customer
_____ e. input

99. Who in a process defines "quality"
_____ a. the customer
_____ b. the supplier
_____ c. the worker
_____ d. management

100. Which of the following is not part of the continuous improvement process?
_____ a. identifying the customer
_____ b. determining what the customer needs and wants
_____ c. providing what the customer wants and improving on that
_____ d. projecting what the customer will want in the future

101. What is the difference between a common variation and a special variation?
_____ a. common variations are normal and controllable while special variations are uncontrollable
_____ b. common variations are random in nature and can not be controlled while special variations are those that are caused by changes in the process

_____ c. special variations are those outside the actual system that have an impact on the system while common variations are within the system

_____ d. none of the above

102. Which of the following contains an item that is not a variable category?

_____ a. machine and methods

_____ b. environment and manpower

_____ c. materials and finance

_____ d. policy and methods

ANSWERS TO CHAPTER 3
QUALITY IMPROVEMENT CONCEPTS
QUESTIONS

1. **c** Deming's 14 points discuss processes, rather than organizational structures, on a continuous process of improvement, and the use of data. One of the fourteen points specifically speaks against management by objectives.

2. **a** The philosophical foundations, or elements, of CQI are customer focus, systems view, data-driven analysis, implementer (owner) involvement, multiple causation, solution identification solution identification, process optimization, continuing improvement, and organizational learning.

3. **b** Shewhart, on of the "founders" of the CQI/TQM approach, has noted that price without an understanding of quality is meaningless, and that a focus on low price would lead to additional expense in the long run.

4. **a** Physicians and employees are the internal customers of a hospital; patients are typically considered external customers. Physicians are considered by most managers as "internal customers essential to any quality improvement initiative," although considering employee satisfaction from the view of employee as customer is a relatively new concept.

5. **d** All of these are considered to be customers in a CQI system, and efforts must be directed to ensure that customer satisfaction is maintained. Probably the newest aspect of a CQI approach is viewing payers (e.g. insurers) as customers that must be satisfied, typically by providing service at the lowest possible cost.

6. **a** A physician, for example, supplies patients (customers) to the hospital, but is also a consumer of its services and must be satisfied on both levels for optimum quality.

7. **b** Although all of these individuals provide valuable information about both process and outcome, the definer of quality is the consumer of services, not the provider (employee/supplier) or the optimizer of processes (manager).

8. **d** In CQI, there is an emphasis on optimizing the delivery process to meet customer needs, regardless of precedents, and to implement system changes, regardless of turf issues.

9. **b** Although all of these are reasons for team failure, as well as jumping to solutions before identifying root causes, lack of rewards and recognition, and a lack of urgency or a champion for the project, the main reason for team failure is lack of effective training.

10. **a** The three phases in the formation and use of CQI teams are *orientation*, which includes establishment of operating procedures, sharing of problem-related information, and presentation of specialized/technical information; *evaluation*, which includes analysis of the problem, generation of alternatives, establishment of evaluation criteria, evaluation of alternatives, and reconciliation of interests; and *control*, which positions group solutions in relation to those acceptable to environmental powers, recommendation of alternatives, and implementation of the plan.

11. **d** All of these might indicate problems in the process of patient transport. A flowchart will show the steps in the process, which might help in identifying the "week link." A cause-effect diagram will help a group or individual in charge of solving a patient transport problem with brainstorming a solution, and the Pareto chart (e.g., of time it takes to complete each step in the process) might identify where the longest delays are occurring.

12. **c** The Pareto principle states that whenever a quality problem has multiple causes, just a few of those causes account for most of the incidents. By using a Pareto chart, which is a histogram that displays the relative frequency of causes, a quality team can determine which problems need to be attacked first.

13. **b** A process is considered under control when most observations are near the centerline, with a few points near both the upper and lower control limits. However, most health care errors tend to be asymmetrical, a consistent observation of points above or below the center can indicate a problem as well.

14. **c** The control limits of a control chart are typically standard deviations.

15. **a** The x-bar chart plots the mean; s-bar, the standard deviation; r-bar, the range; and a p-chart, errors or proportions of success.

16. **a** Run charts serve the function of showing where one is compared with where one has been, and do not specify control limits.

17. **d** A histogram is a bar chart that represents the frequency distribution of a set of data without the ordering seen in a Pareto chart.

18. **a** Continuity of care reflects a consistent standard of care; it would *not* indicate who provides that care. Although one would expect a similar level of training, barring legal mandates, it is not unreasonable to expect that a radiographer could not give injections as long as the training received was consistent. In a CQI setting, *all* employees are considered staff.

19. **c** Unsolicited complaints and telephone hotlines are only good for bringing about lower level understanding of customer needs. Focus groups, benchmarking, personal interviews, and structured surveys will bring about the highest level of understanding of customer needs.

20. **a** Individual variation in response due to predisposition or other biases may influence response (response-set bias); however, variations in response due to time of day, temperature of the room or the presence of others may influence response. For example, poor parking facilities may cause a customer to rate radiology services lower than expected.

21. **a**   The reproducibility of measures describes reliability. Construct validity is the extent to which a measure agrees with others instruments thought to measure the same thing; content validity is the extent to which a survey covers the content area; and criterion validity compares the results of a survey to a criterion measure.

22. **a**   The mean provides the greatest reliability in the three measures of central tendency (mean, median, and mode); the standard deviation is a measure of dispersion.

23. **b**   Whenever a distribution is skewed or incomplete, or if it is most important to determine whether cases fall into upper or lower halves of the distribution and not how far from the central point, the median is calculated.

24. **c**   The mode provides information about the most typical case, but provides only a rough estimate of central value.

25. **d**   The standard deviation will provide interpretive information about the normal distribution curve, and provides information that will be needed if further interpretation and calculations are necessary.

26. **d**   The analysis of variance tests one or more hypotheses indicating that the means of all groups sampled come from populations with equal means, differing only because of sampling error. Simple correlation measures the degree of relationship between two variables.

27. **a**   The range divided by six should be approximately equal to one standard deviation when the sample size is approximately 100.

28. **b**   All this data shows is that more serious reactions exist in the older population. If this is a hospital that serves a primarily geriatric population, fewer reactions among younger patients should be expected, simply because the population of older patients is larger than that of younger patients. The statistical proportion of contrast reactions in the older population may be the same as or even less than that of the younger population. Without further information, only "b" can be seen as correct.

29. **d**   Provider performance is often easy to measure; however, it does not necessarily provide the best information, especially in situations where accepted standards of care do not exist, the technology is new or untested, and great range exists in patient variables.

30. **b**   This is not necessarily a correct assumption; outcomes vary based on inputs (patient population) as well as the process (resources available, provider performance). This is the information that has predominantly been available in databases. For example, a cancer center may be accepting only the sickest patients with little hope of remission or recovery and thus engages in mostly experimental treatments. In such a case, a survival rate of one year is perhaps phenomenal and cannot be compared to a cancer center with a five year survival rate, but has patients that, on the most part, have a reasonable hope of "recovery".

31. **c**   Risk adjustment or severity adjustment allows for better comparison of hospitals in terms of outcomes (report cards); a particular problem for academic health centers who tend to receive the cases with the highest risk and complexity through referral networks or dumping.

32. **d**   Although all of these movements have indicated or reinforced the need for hospitals to be responsible for establishing standards of care, the *Darling vs. Charleston Memorial Hospital* case first established that a hospital governing body must know the standards of care and the actions staff take to resolve them.

33. **d**   Benchmarking seeks to identify the best practices in related and unrelated settings and find ways to emulate best practices or use them as performance standards. Often the emulation of best practices in unrelated settings is the most difficult for health care professionals (e.g., "My patients aren't customers?").

34. **c**   Absolute or normative standards typically come from academic health care centers and through clinical trials; empirical standards are relative to other institutions treating similar patients; and institutional standards are those of the institution. The danger of institutional standards is that the institution uses itself as its own control, whereas absolute standards may be unattainable, and the "average" standard of the community may be misleading, if this level of care is poor.

35. **a** For example, a hospital that does a poor job in coding comorbidities will have an apparent "poor" ranking in relationship to other hospitals, and a hospital that does a good job in coding complications will also have a ranking that appears "poor" in relationship to other hospitals. It must be remembered that data is simply information, and poor or good handling of that information will have definite outcomes on the presentation of that information.

36. **b** All of these individuals are customers due to the fact that they are influenced in their satisfaction by the product (requisition) generated by the admissions desk. However, the individual with the greatest stake is the technologist. Thus, an improperly generated requisition causes extra work for, and decreases the satisfaction of, the staff technologist.

37. **a** Both conformance quality and quality assurance are related to meeting a predetermined set of standards. Requirements quality refers to meeting all the customer's requirements with a product, or providing service that meets or exceeds those requirements. Quality of a kind refers to a product or service that greatly exceeds the customer's requirements. Total quality is a system of continuous improvement.

38. **c** Customer opinion is certainly important (in terms of quality–the most important attribute), and may form one data-set, but determining the cause of a problem requires empirical data.

39. **d** Quality goals must be specifically worded, and vague statements are to be avoided. Instead, according to Juran, they must be phrased in such a way that their achievement (or lack thereof) can be evaluated.

40. b Philip B. Crosby's statement, "quality is free," does not mean that quality does not cost money; in fact achieving quality can be quite expensive. Instead, it means that overall (including hidden costs), the cost of not achieving quality or zero defects can be much more expensive than the obvious costs associated with quality improvement efforts.

41. d These are all components of Crosby's approach to total quality, and the emphasis on hidden costs is usually quite good to illustrate to managers who have not bought into quality improvement how valuable quality can be to their institution, as well as the negative outcomes if they do not seek zero defects.

42. b It can be said that no process is truly problem-free, and CQI works even for processes in which no apparent problems are observed.

43. d Unfortunately, many individuals see CQI as just another quick fix or management fad. In reality, unless the institution is really committed to quality, it might be better to not even attempt CQI. It takes 6–12 months to get people knowledgeable enough to begin planning for CQI; another 6–12 months to complete the first wave of training, and up to 10 years to fully implement CQI.

44. c Although all of these are influenced by medical specialization, communication is the most impacted. It leads to "fiefdoms," individuals who believe that only their area can provide what the customer needs, so they do not speak each other's language. Also, specialization tends to encourage individuals to "learn more and more about less and less."

45. a One thing the empirical studies about CQI have found consistently is that employee job satisfaction increases with the implementation of CQI.

46. b The amount of waste in health care costs is estimated at about 20–40%, which does not include costs such as the cost of clinical errors.

47. a   Too much diversity may mean that teams no longer share common goals, limiting their effectiveness. Some of this can be ameliorated by training in group processes.

48. a   A process owner can either support or hinder the improvement process, and must possess both knowledge of the customer and the task-related knowledge of a process.

49. b   One of the dilemmas of CQI is making professionals understand that situational conflict, which is typically high in any successful organization, is not the same thing as interpersonal conflict. A successful team will be able to manage all types of conflict and help team members differentiate interpersonal from situational conflict.

50. c   The TQM philosophy is based on collective responsibility, accountability, and participation, all of which may conflict with traditionally held notions of professional autonomy.

51. d   TQM recognizes that there is competition to be studied and surpassed, with the customer's experience as the basis of comparison, and the continuous improvement is to be built into the process. To study competition requires comparing one's current performance against that of the competition, known as benchmarking.

52. a   In CQI/TQM, management makes fewer decisions, but instead manages the culture of the organization and allocates resources to support the change process.

53. d   As leaders in health care, especially health care teaching and research, academic health centers need to be involved in CQI and TQM both to teach future leaders about quality, as well as to conduct research that will set standards for health care quality.

54. c   By far the biggest disagreement between CEOs and professional employees, such as physicians, is the need for cost reduction; this can be true even in the managed care setting.

55. **a** The best measure of team performance is quality of work products. Focusing on the amount of time needed to solve the problem, leader performance, and developing a large number of work products reflect a more traditional approach which has not proven to be especially effective.

56. **b** Teams outperform individuals working alone. They may appear to be more costly only if one does not take into account the hidden costs of not achieving quality.

57. **c** Management needs to get out of the way to help a team work, and its best function is to continue to stress the importance of the work effort.

58. **d** In the 1860s, Florence Nightingale used a systematic approach to collecting and analyzing mortality rates in hospitals.

59. **d** A small number of individuals, individuals with complimentary skills, and individuals with a common purpose are all components of effective teams.

60. **d** Cooperating departments with the best intentions often lose sight of subtle slippage in effectiveness and efficiency, seeing those as acceptable post implementation adjustments. Periodic meetings with employees (team members) and managers are useful to provide ongoing critique and assessment. Also, a dedicated individual in the institution should monitor CQI efforts.

61. **c** Long-term purchase contracts might be useful in reducing the cost of direct supplies. Developing critical pathways, improving discharge planning, reducing days lost due to waiting for diagnostic tests, and developing process improvement plans are all ways to reduce the average length of stay.

62. **a** Identifying all customers for each service and development of a CQI panel are both fundamental elements of a well-developed CQI program, along with providing a well-developed vision statement and goals, development of a monitoring group, and stakeholder (including physician) involvement; however, the main job of management in CQI is to optimize the system and then get out of the way.

63. **b**   Although all of the responses discuss or describe portions of the process, the best definition of a process is a series of steps that achieve a desired outcome.

64. **c**   CQI typically requires a lot of training, and the team approach requires a number of meetings to assess and optimize the process. This will cost money. Where CQI should save money is in reducing waste of labor and waste of materials.

65. **a**   Although teams should look at all the data, and assess accordingly, in some cases, one negative event–called a sentinel event–is the component that requires immediate or sole attention.

66. **b**   The Shewhart cycle consists of plan, do check, act (PDCA), and today has been amended to FOCUS-PDCA (find a process to improve, organize to improve the process, clarify current knowledge of the process, understand the sources of process variation, select the process improvement plan, plan the improvement, do the improvement to the process, study the results, and act to hold the gain and continue to improve the process).

67. **a**   In a flowchart, an input or output is represented by an oval; an activity by a rectangle; and a decision by a quadrangle.

68. **c**   Multivoting and rank ordering are used to rank the ideas generated in a group. In multivoting, each member is allowed to vote for 1/3 of the ideas, and in rank ordering all ideas are ranked, with "1" being the most important ideas. In both cases, the ideas with the fewest votes or lowest rankings are eliminated.

69. **d**   Simply adding another layer of "stat" will probably not be helpful, instead what is needed is brainstorming and the collection of data to see why the "stat" designation is so abused.

70. **b** Although the radiologist and patient are certainly customers in the production of a report, the primary customer is the referring physician. The transcriptionist is considered to be the supplier of the service.

71. **d** The insurance company is the supplier of services in this instance. The primary customer is the hospital or radiology department.

72. **c** Employees, known as internal customers, require services from other employees to perform their job. Job dissatisfaction is a factor in making employees less effective in handling customers, particularly in terms of problems they feel unable to control. They also serve a marketing function by serving as representatives of the institution to friends, family, and acquaintances.

73. **d** Although it is often assumed that third-party customers or payers only care about cost, they also expect quality clinical services for their constituent groups, ease of administration, and accurate, timely information. This can be seen, for example, in the "report cards" that have been developed by many payers regarding the efficacy of clinical services by providers.

74. **a** It does cost about 5–10 times more to recruit a new customer than to retain an old one. Most customers will continue to do business with an organization with which they have problems, if the organization attempts to address those problems. Interestingly, complainers are more likely to return to an organization with which they had problems than non-complainers.

75. **d** Training outcomes are measured by a survey following the seminar or training. Any such survey must be based on the criteria established for customer service (based on needs assessment), and should include measurement of changes in attitude, effectiveness, and appropriateness.

76. **d** Although certainly new technology and efficient personnel are important, and may lead to a physician's happiness, the most important thing for any service provider to realize is that physicians value most services that contribute to their ease of practice.

77. **c** The process for correcting customer complaints is known as service recovery. The JCAHO requires accredited institutions to have such a process in place.

78. **b** The patient is the primary customer when visiting the physician and when the technologist performs the examination; the insurance company, or payer, is the customer when the bill is sent to the third-party payer.

79. **c** Although traditionally the supplier has been the referring physician when patients present for radiology services, the ability of patients in many instances to self-refer themselves for mammography services would make them both supplier and customer.

80. **c** Workers who are closest to a problem are the most likely to see and understand their problem.

81. **a** Although profitability and efficiency are some of the desired outcomes of TQM, theory does not predict such an outcome.

82. **a** TQM is a management philosophy that states quality is the ultimate goal of any organization so as to improve the product and increase market share. CQI is the methodology of identifying potential problems, designing possible solutions, collecting data, and analyzing the outcome. CQI is a circular process which repeats itself endlessly.

83. **b** Quality outcomes are the goal of both Quality Assurance and Quality Management. However, QA focuses on setting standards and addressing only those parts of the system that are not within those standards. QM implies that there are no upper levels of quality past which the quality is "good enough."

84. **c** Although one possible focus of an effective organization may be employee rewards, the focus of QI is on the needs of the organization, employees, customers, and supplies.

85. **d** A statistical profile of quality is usually obtained by sampling products as opposed to mass inspections. Because these inspections are retrospective, they are only identifying "problems" and do not add to the quality of the product directly. Such an approach allows individual employees to neglect quality as someone else is responsible for that.

86. **d** In addition to the above, job training should include how a job contributes to the purpose and an operational understanding of others jobs (professions/positions) within the organization.

87. **c** According to Deming, merit rating systems have almost the exact opposite impact of an organization than they are intended to have. The net effect of such a system is reduced quality, reduced employee satisfaction, and lack of cooperation.

88. **a** Unless everyone in an organization understands and takes responsibility for striving to meet the mission, vision, and principles of the organization, it will be impossible to meet them.

89. **d** Vision statements should describe a possible, desirable future, visualize new responsibilities for the organization and the employees, describe how others should see your organization, and define a target to reach. In order to successfully do that, the vision statement should meet all three of the above criteria.

90. **d** All of the listed criteria should include a good mission statement.

91. **b** Guiding principles do not address authority within an organization but do identify core values, incorporate TQM principles, empower employees, and are consistent with the mission and vision statements.

92. **a** For valid and reliable information gathering, a high rate of response is needed. If a questionnaire is only given by an employee, the level of response will fall.

93. **a** Key Quality Characteristics (KQCs) are those aspects or qualities that are most important to the customer. Unless these are constantly measured and improved, customer satisfaction will not increase.

94. **a** Key Process Variable (KPVs) are the components of any process that affect the outcome of the process. Items listed in I above are the components of any system being evaluated.

95. **d** A "customer" is anyone who is affected by the "owner" of a process such as receptionist from whom KQCs can be determined. In this example, the patient is the obvious customer but the technologists receive and act on the results of the receptionist's actions. Physicians are also customers in that their actions are determined, in part, by the actions of the receptionist. As an example, if the receptionist misschedules, delays, or inconveniences, the patient, the timeliness of the physician's actions can also be affected.

96. **d** There are four steps necessary to define and measure quality. The first step is to define the process. The second step is to identify the Key Quality Concepts that need to be measured. The third step is to operationally define the DQCs so that the proper data can be collected. Finally, a data collection plan needs to be created and implemented.

97. **b** An operational definition is one that is so explicit that there is no interpretation necessary to determine if something meets that definition. For example, the definition of "excessive base + fog" might be given as any OD value above .30 when measured with a calibrated densitometer on an area a developed sheet of film that has not been exposed to light or radiation prior to development.

98. **c** The five steps of any simple process are supplier, input, action, output, and customer. A process is that series of actions repeated over and over again in order to transform the inputs into the outputs.

99. **a** According to Deming, it is the customer that determines what constitutes quality. If customers are not satisfied with the end product (output) they will stop using the process and it will cease to exist.

100. **d** In the continuous improvement process, projecting the future is not necessary. As the cycle of identifying the customers and determining what they want and need, the future needs and wants will be incorporated into the system as the customers become aware of them.

101. b   All processes have some level of inherent random variation that cannot be controlled by changing the system. These are outside the control of the system and are referred to as common variations. Special variations are those that are introduced into the system by changing the steps of the system itself.

102. c   The five major categories of variables in specific Key Quality Concepts are manpower (then number and qualification of people in the process), machines (equipment used in the process), materials (the types and quality of materials used in the process), methods (how the machine, manpower, and materials come together to produce the output), environment (physical and psychological aspects of the milieu in which the process occurs), and policies (steps in the procedure and policy manual used in the process).

Quality Improvement Data

MULTIPLE-CHOICE QUESTIONS

1. A chief technologist of a 250-bed hospital radiology department wishes to compare staffing in his hospital with similar hospitals. He surveys 10 other hospitals in his region, finding the following:

	A	B	C	D	E	F	G	H
Number of R/F Rooms	5	4	6	7	5	6	5	5
Number of Technologists	7	8	10	11	8	10	9	9

    What is the mean number of technologists employed?
    ____ a. 5
    ____ b. 5.2
    ____ c. 8
    ____ d. 9

2. In the following data set:

	A	B	C	D	E	F	G	H
Number of R/F Rooms	5	4	6	7	5	6	5	5
Number of Technologists	7	8	10	11	8	10	9	9

    What is the ratio of technologists to rooms, on average (mean)?
    ____ a. 1:1   ____ c. 1.89:1
    ____ b. 1.67:1   ____ d. 2:1

3. In room 1, 2 of every 25 films are repeated. In room 2, it is 3 or every 35. Which room has the lower repeat rate?

   ____ a. room 1
   ____ b. room 2

4. Which of the following is true with a mean score of 80, and a standard deviation of 5.

   I. A score of 85 is one standard deviation above the mean.

   II. A score of 90 is two standard deviations above the mean.

   III. A score of 95 is four standard deviations above the mean.

   ____ a. I and II only
   ____ b. I and III only
   ____ c. II and III only
   ____ d. I, II, and III

5. Although the temperatures in Nome, Alaska and Honolulu, Hawaii over the course of a winter day might be quite disparate, their variance might be similar.

   ____ a. true
   ____ b. false

6. If you gave two surveys of patient satisfaction, and achieved a 90% return on the first set, and 60% on the second set, which of these is a reasonable conclusion?

   ____ a. The second set cannot be trusted.
   ____ b. Both sets are within acceptable parameters for returned surveys.
   ____ c. The second set would most likely provide sampling error.
   ____ d. none of the above

7. A study of your repeat rate for trauma reveals that it is 8.0%. In general radiography, it averages 5.0%. Which of these are reasonable conclusions?
    _____ a. Trauma is probably higher due to patient mix and complexity.
    _____ b. Trauma's rate is unacceptable.
    _____ c. Both rates are unacceptable.
    _____ d. There is probably one "bad" technologist in trauma.

8. The percent of area under the normal curve that is ± one standard deviation from the means is:
    _____ a. 68%
    _____ b. 95%
    _____ c. 99%
    _____ d. 100%

9. Calculate the standard deviation of the following set: 1, 2, 4, 6, 8, 9.
    _____ a. 1.95
    _____ b. 2.95
    _____ c. 3.95
    _____ d. 4.95

10. A large variance in response will most likely have what effect on standard deviation?
    _____ a. It gives a high standard deviation.
    _____ b. It gives a low standard deviation.
    _____ c. It has a moderate effect on standard deviation.
    _____ d. It has no effect on standard deviation.

11. In general, the larger a focus group, the better, as it will provide more chance for input to be statistically significant.
    _____ a. true
    _____ b. false

12. Which of the following typically involves a retro-spective research study?
    _____ a. clinical trials of medications or procedures
    _____ b. review of databases
    _____ c. evaluation of patient outcomes
    _____ d. b and c

13. Which of the following is the minimum of data sets required for reproducibility?
    _____ a. one
    _____ b. two
    _____ c. three
    _____ d. twenty

14. Raymond Jones thinks that the wait times for outpatients in his facility are excessive, having gathered the following data:

Wait Time	% of Patients
>5 min	20
>10 min	30
>15 min	30
>10 min	10
20+ min	10

    His benchmarks are 2 local competitors who guarantee wait times of 15 minutes or less. Which of the following is (are) logical conclusions, based on the above?
    _____ a. His wait times are excessive.
    _____ b. His wait times are acceptable.
    _____ c. He needs more information on how well his competitors comply with their guarantee.
    _____ d. none of the above

15. What is the most likely effect shown in Figure 4-1?
    _____ a. patient communications errors
    _____ b. patient satisfaction
    _____ c. patient noncompliance
    _____ d. missed diagnoses

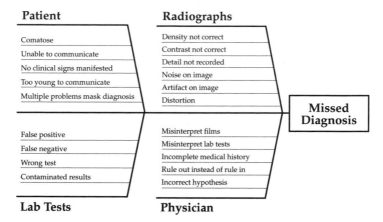

Figure 4-1

16. What is the most likely effect shown in Figure 4-2?
    _____ a. physician problems with radiology
    _____ b. patient problems with radiology
    _____ c. reasons for canceling barium contrast
              examinations
    _____ d. none of the above

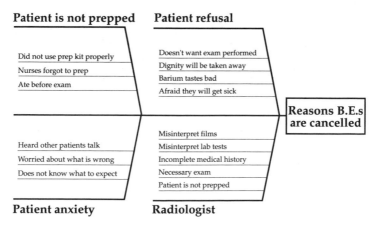

Figure 4-2

17. Which of the following is illustrated in Figure 4-3?
_____ a. histogram   _____ c. run chart
_____ b. Pareto chart   _____ d. scatter diagram

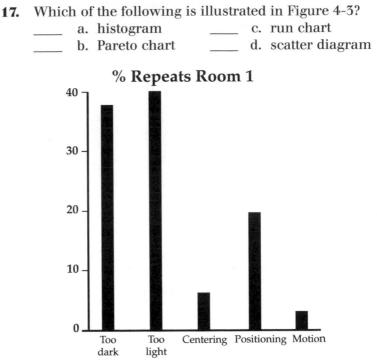

% Repeats Room 1

Figure 4-3

18. Which of the following is most likely true in Figure 4-4?
_____ a. Patient factors caused the most repeats.
_____ b. Machine factors caused the most repeats.
_____ c. Technologist factors caused the most repeats.
_____ d. none of the above

19. Which of the following most likely true regarding Figure 4-5?
_____ a. The inservice was implemented in June.
_____ b. The inservice was implemented in January and a new employee began in August.
_____ c. The zero cases in November are normal random fluctuation.
_____ d. Two of the above are true.

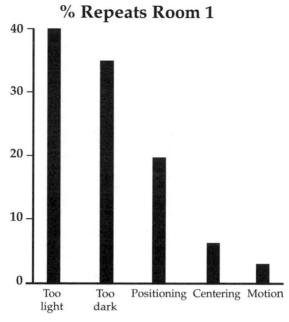

Figure 4-4

Number of Infections
Following Service

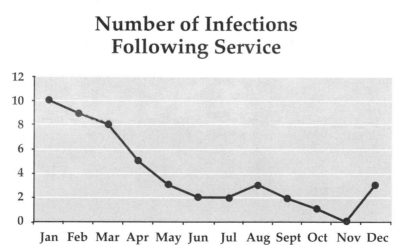

Figure 4-5

20. Which of the following are designed to work with subsystems containing trend charts?

    _____ a. one major variable

    _____ b. two major variables

    _____ c. three or four major variables

    _____ d. any number of major variables

21. What is the purpose of a trend chard?

    _____ a. It shows how well you are doing.

    _____ b. It shows failure.

    _____ c. It sustains quality

    _____ d. all of the above

22. A system in control should show no variation.

    _____ a. true

    _____ b. false

23. Which of the following is not a clue on a trend chart that a system is out of control?

    _____ a. three or more points on the target line

    _____ b. three or more points at the limit

    _____ c. three points above or below the target line

    _____ d. a majority of data points on one side of the target line

24. Which of the following are reasons, from a trend chart, to suspect that your system is out of control.

    _____ a. Three data points exceed one standard deviation.

    _____ b. Three data points exceed two standard deviations.

    _____ c. Five data points exceed two standard deviations.

    _____ d. Five data points exceed two standard deviations.

25. What is the definition of a histogram?

    _____ a. a variance in the system over time

    _____ b. a bar graph showing the frequency vs. time

    _____ c. an assessment of central tendencies over time

    _____ d. all of the above

26. Which of the following sets contains variables that do *not* lend themselves to histograms?
    I.   patient waiting time, patient time of day, patient types of exams
    II. disease population, workload by hour, exam value
    III. procedure type of hours, computer down time, number of incomplete requests by unit

    ____ a. I and II only
    ____ b. I and III only
    ____ c. II and III only
    ____ d. I, II, and III

27. At which interval on Figure 4-6 is the mode?
    ____ a. A
    ____ b. B
    ____ c. C
    ____ d. D

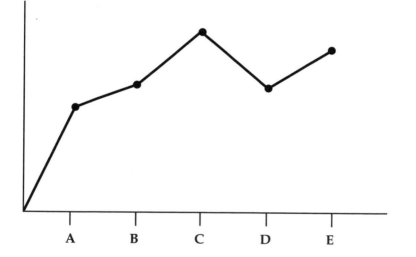

Figure 4-6

28. What is the relationship of the value to the baseline at point 'E' of Figure 4-7?

_____ a. higher
_____ b. lower
_____ c. same
_____ d. not enough information

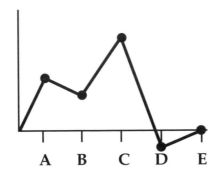

A   B   C   D   E

Figure 4-7

29. What is the name of the type of graph shown in Figure 4-8?

_____ a. scattergram
_____ b. point graph
_____ c. matrix graph
_____ d. linear graph

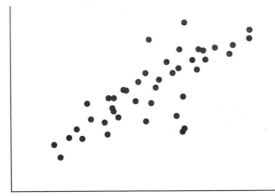

Figure 4-8

30. What is the definition of a false positive?
_____ a. something that is true but the test shows it to be not true
_____ b. something that is false but the test shows it to be true
_____ c. something that is true and the test shows it to be true
_____ d. something that is false and test shows it to be not true

31. What is sensitivity?
_____ a. the ability to detect values close to zero
_____ b. the ability to detect very small changes in values
_____ c. the size of the units used by the instrument
_____ d. the range of values the instrument can measure

32. Which statement best differentiates reliability and accuracy?
_____ a. Reliability is getting the correct information and accuracy has to do with how often the information is correct.
_____ b. Reliability is the ability of an instrument to detect and accuracy has to do with how correct that information is.
_____ c. Reliability is how correct the information is and accuracy has to do with how faithful it is to reality.
_____ d. Reliability is always getting the same value from the same conditions and accuracy has to do with how correct that value is.

33. What is inter-observer reliability?
_____ a. The same observer always give the same observation.
_____ b. All observers give different values for the same situation.
_____ c. The variation in values between observers is acceptably low.
_____ d. none of the above

34. What is the definition of correlation?
    ____ a. cause-and-effect
    ____ b. precursor and event
    ____ c. events tend to occur at the same time
    ____ d. none of the above

35. What is the most common way to diagram factors that cause variability in a system?
    ____ a. line graph
    ____ b. cause-and-effect diagram
    ____ c. flow chart
    ____ d. none of the above

36. What is another name for the Pareto Chart?
    ____ a. bar graph
    ____ b. scatter graph
    ____ c. line graph
    ____ d. flow chart

37. What term describes the result of actions under ideal circumstances or results, and usual or normal circumstances?
    ____ a. efficacy
    ____ b. efficiency
    ____ c. effectiveness
    ____ d. all of the above

38. What requires a consideration of outcomes but does not require consideration of the cost of the action?
    ____ a. efficacy
    ____ b. efficiency
    ____ c. effectiveness
    ____ d. all of the above

39. Which of the following describes the quality of an output achieved for a given level of input?
    ____ a. efficacy
    ____ b. efficiency
    ____ c. effectiveness
    ____ d. all of the above

40. What term describes the distribution and types of patients cared for in a health facility?
    ____ a. epidemiology
    ____ b. case mix
    ____ c. outpatient care
    ____ d. case mix index

41. What term describes the amount by which the cost of treating the average Medicare patient in a hospital varies from the comparable cost for all hospitals?
    ____ a. epidemiology
    ____ b. case mix
    ____ c. outpatient care
    ____ d. case mix index

42. Which of the following is defined by the JCAHO as a measurement tool to monitor the quality of an indicator?
    ____ a. important governance functions
    ____ b. management
    ____ c. clinical functions
    ____ d. all of the above

43. Which of the following is true according to JCAHO regarding an incident?
    I.   applies to patients only
    II. causes harm
    III. has the potential to cause harm

    ____ a. I and II only
    ____ b. I and III only
    ____ c. II and III only
    ____ d. I, II, and III

44. Which of the following describes quality management?
    ____ a. A management activity aimed at improving effectiveness.
    ____ b. A management activity aimed at improving efficiency.
    ____ c. A management activity that is ongoing.
    ____ d. all of the above

45. Which of the following is the goal of benchmarking?
____ a. to be the best in the business
____ b. to know the limits
____ c. to show patients you are as good as other hospitals
____ d. all of the above

46. Which of the following are included by JCAHO under "doing the right thing?"
I.   efficacy
II. appropriateness
III. availability

____ a. I and II only
____ b. I and III only
____ c. II and III only
____ d. I, II, and III

47. What term describes the degree to which care for the patient is coordinated, over time, among practitioners and organizations.
____ a. efficiency   ____ c. continuity
____ b. efficacy   ____ d. appropriateness

48. What term describes the characteristics of what is done and how it is done?
____ a. efficacy
____ b. appropriateness
____ c. safety
____ d. dimensions of performance

49. Which of the following are uninterpreted observations or facts?
____ a. functions   ____ c. information
____ b. data   ____ d. assessments

50. Which of the following describes the degree to which the risk of an intervention and the risk in the care environment are reduced for the patient and others, including health care providers?
____ a. timeliness   ____ c. efficiency
____ b. efficacy   ____ d. safety

ANSWERS TO CHAPTER 4
QUALITY IMPROVEMENT DATA QUESTIONS

1. c   The mean is obtained by adding up a set of scores and dividing by the number of scores. Adding up the number of technologists gives 72, and there are 9 scores; 72 divided by 9 is 8.

2. b   The mean number of rooms is 4.78 (43 divided by 9); the mean number of technologists is 8. To calculate the ratio of technologists to rooms, divide 8 by 4.78, which gives 1.67.

3. b   The repeat rate is calculated by dividing the number of necessary repeats by the total number of films, thus: $2 \div 25 = 0.08$ or 8%, and $3 \div 35 = 0.086$ or 8.6%. Room 2 has a slightly higher repeat rate.

4. a   Each increment of 5 is one standard deviation above or below the mean; thus a score of 70 is two standard deviations below the mean; 75 is one standard deviation below the mean; 85 is one standard deviation above the mean; and 90 is two standard deviations below the mean.

5. a   Even though it may be very cold in Nome, and pleasantly warm in Hawaii, the variance (the amount the temperature varies) could be similar or even identical for both.

6. c   Since the original sample size is not known, it cannot be determined whether a sufficient sample exists in either case; however, the second set is more likely to produce sampling error.

7. a   The most reasonable conclusion is that trauma has a higher repeat rate due to patient mix and complexity. Whether one or either rate is acceptable depends on a number of factors, and jumping to the conclusion that it must be one "bad" technologist is counterproductive, and not consistent with a CQI approach.

8. a   The percent of area under the normal curve is ± 1 standard deviation from the mean is 68%, within ± 2 standard deviations is 95%, within ± 3 standard deviations is 99%, and within ± 6 standard deviations is almost 100%.

9. b Standard deviation is the square root of the sum of the squared deviations from the mean divided by the total number of scores. The mean of this set is 5; thus, for example 9–5 = 4, and 4 squared is 16; 8–5 = 3, and 3 squared is 9, and so on. The sum of all the squares is 52, when that is divided by the total number of scores, we get 8.67, and the square root of 8.67 is 2.95.

10. a Standard deviation is an easily, algebraically manipulated measure of variability; thus increases in variability or variance will increase standard deviation proportionally.

11. b A focus group is best seen as a type of team, and teams do not follow the same rules as one would make for a survey. In general, some diversity is needed, but excessive diversity could lead to lack of common goals or viewpoints, which could limit the team's effectiveness.

12. d Clinical trials are typically prospective (future-based) studies, whereas epidemiologic, database, and outcome evaluations are typically retrospective studies.

13. c The minimum number of data sets required for reproducibility is three, with some sources recommending five or ten. Typically more are required to document a service problem than for routine QC.

14. c Benchmarking is not simply comparing numbers; it is also looking at how those numbers are achieved. A visit or call to other administrators would be helpful here.

15. d In this cause-and-effect or fishbone diagram, in the box on the right, the effect is missed diagnoses.

16. c In this cause-and-effect or fishbone diagram, in the box on the right, the effect is reasons for canceling barium contrast examinations.

17. a This unordered bar chart is a histogram. Pareto charts are similar, but show the data from the longest bar on the left to the shortest on the right.

18. **c** Patient factors (e.g., motion) are not the most likely cause of repeats from this Pareto chart. It is unlikely that a machine fluctuates from light to dark; thus, technologist factors are the most likely cause of repeats here.

19. **d** The inservice was implemented in January and took some time to take hold; a new employee starting in August caused the rate to increase slightly; the zero cases in November represent normal random fluctuation.

20. **c** Trend charts are designed to work with subsystems containing three or four major variables. Major variables are assignable and cause major movement; minor variables are unassignable and fluctuate randomly.

21. **c** The goal of a trend chart is not to show how well you are doing or to show failure; it is designed to prevent failure by providing clues. This helps to sustain quality rather than working to fix a process after failure.

22. **b** Even a system under the best control will show a random distribution of values with numbers that stray to the high and low ends.

23. **c** According to McKinney (1997), the following are all indicators that a system is out of control: any one data point beyond a limit; any pattern over time; sawtooth patterns that move up or down over five days or longer; five consecutive data points all above or below the target line; three or more consecutive points at the limit; three or more points on the target line; three data points exceeding two standard deviations with two points on one side; five consecutive points increasing or decreasing (three for MQSA); majority of points on one side; if five data points exceed one s.d. with four on one side; a wave pattern; or no change after a change in a major variable.

24. **d** According to McKinney (1997), the following are all indicators that a system is out of control: any one data point beyond a limit; any pattern over time; sawtooth patterns that move up or down over five days or longer; five consecutive data points all above or below the target line; three or more consecutive points at the limit; three or more points on the target line; three data points exceeding two standard deviations with two points on one side; five consecutive points increasing or decreasing (three MQSA); majority of points on one side, if five data points exceed one s.d. with four on one side; a wave pattern; or no change after a change in a major variable.

25. **b** The proper term for a "bar graph" is histogram. They graph frequency (at the height of the bar) over time or by other subset such as exam type.

26. **b** The value of an exam and the population of a disease are not frequency over time or subsets and would not lend themselves to a bar graph.

27. **c** The mode is the value that has the highest frequency or number or is the most common value. It is one of the central tendencies of mean (average), mode (most common), and medium (half of the scores are above and half below).

28. **c** When a graph has a vertical (X) axis that goes above and below the horizontal (Y) axis, values are either positive (greater than the baseline), on the horizontal axis (even to the baseline), or negative (below the horizontal axis).

29. **a** A scattergram is used to give a visual presentation of the relationship of values along a two dimensional axis. The purpose of the scattergram is to give visual clues about possible relationships. As an example, the scattergram in this Figure shows that there is a tendency for the values on the vertical axis to increase as the values on the horizontal axis increase.

30. **b** The above choices are the four possible outcomes from any test or evaluation. The actual situation may either be acceptable/true or the situation may be unacceptable/false. Any test on the situation may show the condition to be acceptable/true or it may show the situation to be unacceptable/false. The graph in this Figure shows the possible combinations.

31. b   Sensitive is related to the ability to detect small changes in values. With a high level of sensitivity, values close to zero should be detected but the sensitivity relates to detecting values throughout the range. The units used by the instrument and the minimum/maximum values of the instrument are related to the range.

32. d   Reliability and accuracy are related terms but have different meanings. Reliability means getting the same value in the same situation each time. For example, if a thermometer always read 5° low, it is reliable as it always gives the same information in the same situation. Accuracy has to do with how correct the information is. In the above example, the thermometer is reliable but it is not accurate. It is possible to have a reliable instrument that is not accurate but not to have an accurate instrument that is not reliable.

33. c   Inter-observer, or inter-rater, reliability is a measure of the amount of variation among observers looking at the same situation. In order for quality assessments to be made, that level of variation must be kept to an acceptable, low limit. An example of where a high level of inter-observer variance (low reliability) is evaluation of the maximum number of line/pairs visible on a test radiograph. As everyone's eyes vary, and different people have different operational definitions of what a visible line/pair is, the results will have low reliability.

34. c   Correlations are comparisons between two events or values. A correlation in no way explains cause-and-effect, nor does it indicate a precursor and event. A correlation only indicates that when one thing happens, something else tends to happen or not happen. Correlation can be direct/positive where one value goes up and the other goes up. Or it can be indirect/negative where one value goes up, the other goes down. An example is that there is a negative correlation between the number of trees in an area and the crime rate. There is no cause-and-effect between trees and the crime rate nor is one a precursor for the other. The correlation is due to the fact that the crime rate is very low in the middle of a forest and much higher in the middle of a city where there are few trees.

35. **b** A cause-and-effect (sometimes called a fishbone diagram) is the most common method of diagraming factors that effect a system. Below is a simple fishbone diagram on patient waiting times in radiology.

36. **a** The Pareto Chart is the name given to a specific type of bar graph where the frequency (number) of variations is graphed against the types of variations. An example of this chart is to graph the number of repeated examinations by reason for the repeat.

37. **a** The result of actions under ideal circumstances or results under usual or normal circumstances defines efficacy.

38. **c** Effectiveness requires a consideration of outcomes but does not require consideration of the cost of the action.

39. **b** Effectiveness describes the quality of an output achieved for a given level of input.

40. **b** Case mix is the distribution and types of patients cared for in a health facility. Age, type of illness, source of payment, and acuity are some of the factors that affect case mix.

41. **d** The case mix index is the amount by which the cost of treating the average Medicare patient in a hospital varies from the comparable cost for all hospitals. A number greater than one indicates a more complex case mix than the average, with most hospitals falling between .8000 and 1.200.

42. **d** The JCAHO defines indicator as a measurement tool to monitor the quality of important governance, management, clinical, and support functions.

43. **c** According to JCAHO, an incident is any event in a hospital or other health-care facility that is harmful, may result in injury, that results in an unexpected outcome, or that could cause liability.

44. **d** Quality management is a management activity aimed at improving effectiveness and efficiency. It is an ongoing and continuous process.

45. **a** The goal of benchmarking is to be the best in the business and to surpass all competitive organizations.

46. **a** Both efficacy (the degree to which the care of the patient has been shown to accomplish the desired or projected outcome) and appropriateness (the degree to which care provided is relevant to the patient's clinical needs, given the current state of knowledge) are included under "doing the right thing." Availability (the degree to which appropriate care is available to meet patients' needs) is included under "doing the right thing well."

47. **c** The degree to which care for the patient is coordinated among practitioners, organizations, and over time describes continuity, according to JCAHO.

48. **d** Dimensions of performance are the characteristics of what is done and how it is done.

49. **b** Uninterpreted observations or facts are data; information is interpreted sets of data; organized data that can assist in decision-making.

50. **d** Safety is the degree to which the risk of an intervention in the health care environment is reduced for the patient and others, including health care providers.

Physical Principles

MULTIPLE-CHOICE QUESTIONS

1. Which of the following describes waves that are totally in phase with the resultant composite waveform?
   ____ a. decreased amplitude
   ____ b. increased amplitude
   ____ c. the amplitude of the highest waveform
   ____ d. the amplitude of the lowest waveform

2. In a three-phase, sic-pulse generator at 80 kVp, what is the lowest voltage across the x-ray tube in theory?
   ____ a. 0 kV
   ____ b. 40 kV
   ____ c. 69 kV
   ____ d. 80 kV

3. The type of generator where the AC voltage waveforms are rectified and then fed into a DC frequency modulator is:
   ____ a. single-phase
   ____ b. three-phase, six-pulse
   ____ c. three-phase, twelve-pulse
   ____ d. high-frequency

4. Which of the following is the ideal voltage ripple?
   ____ a. 100%
   ____ b. 13.5%
   ____ c. 3.5%
   ____ d. 0%

5. Which of the following comprises most anode disks for diagnostic radiography equipment?
   ____ a. tungsten
   ____ b. rhenium
   ____ c. molybdenum
   ____ d. all of the above

6. What is the typical anode disk diameter range?
   ____ a. 2.5 cm (1 in)–10 cm (4 in)
   ____ b. 2.5 cm (1 in)–12.5 cm (5 in)
   ____ c. 5 cm (2 in)–10 cm (4 in)
   ____ d. 5 cm (2 in)–12.5 cm (5 in)

7. Which of the following is true if the tilt angle of the anode is near 0?
   ____ a. The actual focal spot will be larger than the effective focal spot.
   ____ b. The effective focal spot will be larger than the actual focal spot.
   ____ c. The effective focal spot will be equal to the actual focal spot.
   ____ d. The above does not provide enough information to determine the relationship between effective and actual focal spot size.

8. What occurs if the tilt angle of the anode is increased?
   ____ a. The size of the actual focal spot increases.
   ____ b. The size of the effective focal spot increases.
   ____ c. The size of the actual focal spot decreases.
   ____ d. The size of the effective focal spot decreases.

9. Poor screen-film contact tends to be more common in which cassettes?
   ____ a. smaller
   ____ b. larger
   ____ c. slower
   ____ d. faster

10. What is the actual cause of blurring in poor screen-film contact?
    ____ a. motion of the light produced in the screen
    ____ b. increased divergence of light
    ____ c. increased distance of the part from the film
    ____ d. none of the above

11. What effect does fog have on the manifest image?
    ____ a. base + fog increases, contrast increases
    ____ b. base + fog increases, contrast decreases
    ____ c. base + fog decreases, contrast decreases
    ____ d. base + fog decreases, contrast increases

12. The lesser-exposed side of the sensitometric strip is fed into the processor first to minimize which of the following?
    ____ a. bromide drag
    ____ b. the time the strip is in the processor
    ____ c. electron activation
    ____ d. chemical contamination

13. Which of the following might be expected as a result of slight contamination of developer with fixer?
    ____ a. increased speed and decreased contrast
    ____ b. decreased speed and increased contrast
    ____ c. increased speed and increased contrast
    ____ d. decreased speed and decreased contrast

14. When the slope of the straight-line portion of the $D_{LOG}E$ curve is greater. Which of the following describes the film in comparisons to other films?
    ____ a. It would be faster.
    ____ b. It would be slower.
    ____ c. It would have lower contrast.
    ____ d. It would have higher contrast.

15. When the plotted curve of a film is "more to the left" or closer to the Y axis, which of the following best describes it in comparison to other films?
   ____ a. It would be faster
   ____ b. It would be slower.
   ____ c. It would have lower contrast.
   ____ d. It would have higher contrast.

16. What is the optical density range of unexposed processed x-ray film?
   ____ a. 0–0.5
   ____ b. 0.1–0.15
   ____ c. 0.5–0.1
   ____ d. 0.15–0.2

17. What is the approximate light transmission rate through unexposed, processed x-ray film?
   ____ a. 100%
   ____ b. 90%
   ____ c. 80%
   ____ d. 70%

18. What is the average gradient range of most radiographic films?
   ____ a. 1.0–2.5
   ____ b. 1.5–3.5
   ____ c. 2.5–3.0
   ____ d. 2.5–3.5

19. What term describes the slope of the tangent at any point on the $D_{LOG}E$ curve?
   ____ a. gradient
   ____ b. speed
   ____ c. D_{max}
   ____ d. D_{min}

20. What term describes a film with a wider range of exposures in the useful density range?
   ____ a. less latitude
   ____ b. greater latitude
   ____ c. more density
   ____ d. less density

21. At what point is D_{max} observed in the $D_{LOG}E$ curve?
    ____ a. gradient   ____ c. toe
    ____ b. latitude   ____ d. shoulder

22. On which of the following will spectral matching have an effect?
    I.   density
    II. contrast
    III. latitude

    ____ a. I and II only
    ____ b. I and III only
    ____ c. II and III only
    ____ d. I, II, and III

23. What is the control value acceptance limit for base + fog in mammography?
    ____ a. 0.01   ____ c. 0.1
    ____ b. 0.03   ____ d. 0.3

24. What is the proper range of temperatures for processing chemical storage?
    ____ a. 40–60° F
    ____ b. 50–60° F
    ____ c. 60–70° F
    ____ d. 70–80° F

25. What term describes the slope of the straight line portion of a $D_{LOG}E$ curve?
    ____ a. D_{max}
    ____ b. shoulder
    ____ c. average gradient
    ____ d. toe

26. The following sensitometry OD readings were made using a 21-step penetrometer: step 8 = .035; step 9 = 0.55; step 12 = 1.95; step 13 = 2.12; and step 14 = 2.78. How would density difference (DD) be calculated?
    ____ a. subtract step 14 from step 8
    ____ b. subtract step 13 from step 8
    ____ c. subtract 14 from step 9
    ____ d. subtract step 13 from step 9

27. Which of the following is (are) true about using a molybdenum as a target material in mammography?
    _____ a. more low energy photons are produced
    _____ b. production of specific x-ray energies required for breast imaging
    _____ c. increased patient dose
    _____ d. all of the above

28. What percent of the beam will be composed of bremsstrahlung with a tungsten target, at 80 kVp?
    _____ a. 100%
    _____ b. 90%
    _____ c. 70%
    _____ d. 50%

29. Comparing emission spectrum graph A (Figure 5–1) to the other graphs, which demonstrates increasing the "Z" number of the target?
    _____ a. graph B   _____ d. graph E
    _____ b. graph C   _____ e. graph F
    _____ c. graph D

30. Comparing emission spectrum Graph A (Figure 5–1) to the other charts, which demonstrates reducing the mAs?
    _____ a. graph B   _____ d. graph E
    _____ b. graph C   _____ e. graph F
    _____ c. graph D

31. Comparing emission spectrum Graph A (Figure 5–1) to the other charts, which demonstrates reducing the kVp?
    _____ a. graph B   _____ d. graph E
    _____ b. graph C   _____ e. graph F
    _____ c. graph D

32. Comparing emission spectrum Graph A (Figure 5–1) to the other charts, which demonstrates a reduction in filtration?
    _____ a. graph B   _____ d. graph E
    _____ b. graph C   _____ e. graph F
    _____ c. graph D

Radiation Distribution Curves

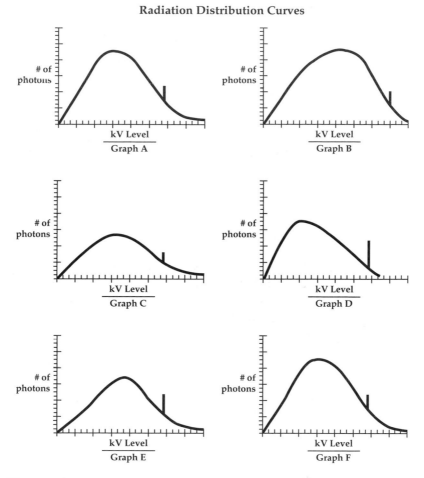

Figure 5-1

33. Comparing emission spectrum of three phase production in Graph A (Figure 5–1) to the other charts, which demonstrates single phase production?

_____ a. graph B
_____ b. graph C
_____ c. graph D
_____ d. graph E
_____ e. graph F

34. Of the following generators, which would have the highest amplitude on the x-ray emission spectrum?
_____ a. high-frequency
_____ b. three-phase
_____ c. single-phase
_____ d. all of the above would have the same amplitude

35. Which of the following are true about the dryer system in an automatic processor?
I. Tubes used have a slit for air to exit.
II. A common temperature would be about 120° F.
III. The duct to the outside should be as straight as possible.

_____ a. I and II only
_____ b. I and III only
_____ c. II and III only
_____ d. I, II, and III

36. Chemical deposits are more likely to form on crossover racks.
_____ a. true
_____ b. false

37. What term describes the first set of rollers in many processors that the film comes into contact within an automatic film processor that is designed to activate the replenishment system?
_____ a. entrance rollers
_____ b. detection rack
_____ c. feed rack
_____ d. all of the above

38. Unexposed silver halide crystals are completely unaffected by the developer.
_____ a. true
_____ b. false

39. Which of the following would be considered to be corrosion-resistant materials for the purposes of mixing and storing processor chemistry?

I. enamel

II. polypropylene

III. aluminum

_____ a. I and II only   _____ c. II and III only

_____ b. I and III only   _____ d. I, II, and III

40. Which is the correct order of the assemblies in an automatic processor?

_____ a. entrance roller, racks, crossovers, turn-arounds, squeegees, dryer

_____ b. entrance roller, racks, turnarounds, crossovers, squeegees, dryer

_____ c. entrance roller, turnarounds, racks, crossovers, dryer, squeegee

_____ d. entrance roller, squeegee, racks, turn-arounds, crossovers, dryer

41. Uniformly mixing the processing and replenisher solutions, maintaining proper temperature and chemical activity, and keeping thoroughly mixed and agitated solutions in constant contact with the films is accomplished by which of the following?

_____ a. transport system

_____ b. water system

_____ c. recirculation system

_____ d. replenishment system

42. To be used for processing, the water supply must be drinkable.

_____ a. true

_____ b. false

43. What method of silver recovery uses iron, usually in the form of steel wool?

_____ a. electrolytic recovery

_____ b. chemical precipitation

_____ c. reverse osmosis

_____ d. metallic replacement

44. What term describes the focal spot size as set by the manufacturer?
    _____ a. normal
    _____ b. nominal
    _____ c. resolution
    _____ d. small

45. What term describes the byproducts that, when allowed to accumulate in large amounts, will act as a barrier to the developer solution?
    _____ a. pi marks
    _____ b. reaction particles
    _____ c. free radicals
    _____ d. solution inhibitors

46. What determines the size of the effective focal spot?
    I.   actual focal spot size
    II. target angle
    III. kVp

    _____ a. I and II only
    _____ b. I and III only
    _____ c. II and III only
    _____ d. I, II, and III

47. Which of the following affect resolution?
    I.   screen speed
    II. screen-film contact
    III. kVp

    _____ a. I and II only
    _____ b. I and III only
    _____ c. II and III only
    _____ d. I, II, and III

48. Spectral matching is the process of ensuring that the set kVp matches the expected emission spectrum.
    _____ a. true
    _____ b. false

49. Which of the following have an effect on radiograph contrast?

I.   film

II. screens

III. focal spot size

_____ a. I and II only

_____ b. I and III only

_____ c. II and III only

_____ d. I, II, and III

50. A technique of 200 mA and .1 sec generated an exposure of 60 mR. What is the mR/mAs?

_____ a. 60

_____ b. 20

_____ c. 12

_____ d. 3

51. Which of the following is (are) true regarding exposures in mammography?

_____ a. Too short of a time of exposure is not problematic.

_____ b. Too long of a time of exposure may cause reciprocity law failure.

_____ c. Exposure times will be fairly consistent for breasts compressed to the same size.

_____ d. two of the above

52. Which of the following is (are) true about mammography exposures?

_____ a. Backup times may be reached due to the inability of the set kVp to penetrate the breast.

_____ b. AECs can be designed to compensate for reciprocity law failure during long exposures.

_____ c. Many new machines have circuits that adjust the kVp to a higher level by sensing the exposure in the first 100 milliseconds.

_____ d. all of the above

53. Which of the following is (are) true regarding mammography?
_____ a. The anode end of the tube is placed directly over the chest wall side of the image to take advantage of the prominent heel effect of the anode.
_____ b. Due to the line-focus principle, resolution is decreased at the chest wall.
_____ c. The actual focal spot and central ray must be placed over the center of the image to compensate for the line focus principle.
_____ d. all of the above

54. Which of the following is (are) an advantage(s) of using rhodium (atomic # = 45) over molybdenum (atomic # = 42) for mammography tube targets?
_____ a. It provides energies for a few keV above molybdenum.
_____ b. It allows for longer exposure times.
_____ c. It is useful for all breast sizes.
_____ d. all of the above

55. What is the minimum HVL on a mammography unit?
_____ a. 0.2 mm Al eq
_____ b. 0.3 mm Al eq
_____ c. 2.0 mm Al eq
_____ d. 2.5 mm Al eq

56. Which of the following describes the process where one filament wire is used for both large and small focal spots and a negative voltage is applied to reduce the size of the electron stream?
_____ a. double focusing
_____ b. grid focusing
_____ c. bias focusing
_____ d. line focusing

57. Which of the following are common methods of measuring contrast in diagnostic radiography?
_____ a. gamma
_____ b. average gradient
_____ c. middle gradient
_____ d. all of the above

58. What would the average gradient be if D2 is 2.2, D1 is 0.45, E2 is 1.2, and E1 is 0.6?
_____ a. 1.47
_____ b. 1.75
_____ c. 2.65
_____ d. 2.92

59. The $D_{LOG}E$ curve of film 1 shows on E1 of 0.8, and an E2 of 1.5. The H&D curve of film 2 shows an E1 of 0.6 and and an E2 of 1.5. Which of the following is a true statement?
_____ a. Both films will have an equal effect on subject contrast.
_____ b. Film 1 will exaggerate subject contrast more than film 2.
_____ c. Film 2 will exaggerate subject contrast more than film 1.
_____ d. none of the above

60. Which of the following is (are) true about the processing chemical hydroquinone?
_____ a. It controls the toe of the curve.
_____ b. It is the primary controller of contrast.
_____ c. It is considered to be a stronger agent.
_____ d. all of the above

61. Which of the following is (are) true about the processing chemical phenidone?
_____ a. It is fast working.
_____ b. It controls the grays of the image.
_____ c. It is the primary controller of sensitivity of the film.
_____ d. all of the above

62. Sensitometers are useful in the comparison of different types of radiographic film.

_____ a. true
_____ b. false

63. Which of the following will be exaggerated if a film has an average gradient above 1?

_____ a. subject contrast
_____ b. gross density
_____ c. image size
_____ d. film-screen contact

64. Increasing the time or temperature of development will have which of the following effects?

I. decrease average gradient
II. increase film speed
III. increase fog

_____ a. I and II only
_____ b. I and III only
_____ c. II and III only
_____ d. I, II, and III

65. Which of the following can be expressed in numeric terms?

I. average gradient
II. speed
III. latitude

_____ a. I and II only
_____ b. I and III only
_____ c. II and III only
_____ d. I, II, and III

66. What term describes a film with a dye added to enable it to better absorb light in the red spectrum?

_____ a. orthochromatic
_____ b. panchromatic
_____ c. high speed
_____ d. slow speed

67. Which of the following represents a doubling of the relative exposure on a $D_{LOG}E$ curve?

_____ a. 0.1
_____ b. 0.3
_____ c. 1.0
_____ d. 3.0

68. If a 100-speed film is represented logarithmically by 2.0, how is a 200-speed film be represented logarithmically?

_____ a. 2.0   _____ c. 3.0
_____ b. 2.3   _____ d. 3.3

69. Which of the following is the minimum quantity of fixer capable of contaminating a 1 gallon developer tank?

_____ a. 2 ml
_____ b. 4 ml
_____ c. 20 ml
_____ d. 40 ml

70. On occasion, your chest unit appears to be "shooting dark." At first, technologists responded by halving density, which produces a light film on the next exposure. Service personnel have found nothing wrong with the unit. This problem only occurs around shift change at 4 PM. Which of the following is the most plausible explanation?

_____ a. Someone is loading the cassettes with wrong speed film.
_____ b. The processor chemicals are depleted.
_____ c. There is probably a fluctuation in the electrical supply
_____ d. Any of the above may explain the problem.

71. What is the typical resolving power of a medium speed intensifying screen?

_____ a. 1 lp/mm
_____ b. 3-10 lp/mm
_____ c. 30-100 lp/mm
_____ d. 100-300 lp/mm

72. Which of the following best describes high average gradient films?

_____ a. high contrast, high speed, and wide latitude

_____ b. high contrast, high speed, and narrow latitude

_____ c. low contrast, low speed, and wide latitude

_____ d. low contrast, low speed, and narrow latitude

73. What term describes the region of image reversal once the $D_{LOG}E$ curve passes D_{max}?

_____ a. gamma

_____ b. gradient

_____ c. solarization

_____ d. antihalation

74. Which of the following are advantages of using greater SIDs?

I.   less magnification

II. decreased patient exposure

III. less tube loading

_____ a. I and II only

_____ b. I and III only

_____ c. II and III only

_____ d. I, II, and III

75. Which of the following are characteristics of single-emulsion films over double-emulsion films?

_____ a. faster speed

_____ b. lower contrast

_____ c. narrow latitude

_____ d. poorer recorded detail

76. What process is designed to prevent the loss of recorded detail in single-emulsion film?

_____ a. gradation

_____ b. halation

_____ c. antigradiation

_____ d. antihalation

77. Which $D_{LOG}E$ curve appears as the "opposite" of radiographic film (i.e., large exposures = lower densities)?

_____ a. cine film

_____ b. single emulsion film

_____ c. duplicating film

_____ d. t-grain film

78. Which of the following are reducing agent in the x-ray film developer?

I.   hydroquinone

II. metol

III. phenidone

_____ a. I only   _____ c. II and III only

_____ b. I and II only   _____ d. I, II, and III

79. What is the proper pH of the developer solution?

_____ a. acidic

_____ b. basic

_____ c. pH variable

_____ d. none of the above

80. What is the proper pH of the fixer solution?

_____ a. acidic

_____ b. basic

_____ c. pH variable

_____ d. none of the above

81. Which chemical is responsible for the rapid development of the gray tones of the radiograph?

_____ a. phenidone

_____ b. aluminum chloride

_____ c. ammonium thiosulfate

_____ d. hydroquinone

82. Which chemical is responsible for development of the black tones of the radiograph?

_____ a. phenidone

_____ b. aluminum chloride

_____ c. ammonium thiosulfate

_____ d. hydroquinone

83. What is the function of chelates in the developer?
_____ a. controls pH
_____ b. maintains chemical concentrations
_____ c. controls for metallic ions
_____ d. all of the above

84. What is the function of acetate in the fixer?
_____ a. maintains pH
_____ b. controls oxidation
_____ c. buffers the water bath
_____ d. all of the above

85. If 100% of the light is transmitted, what will be the OD?
_____ a. 0
_____ b. 0.3
_____ c. 1.0
_____ d. 4.0

86. Which of the following does *not* control image quality and brightness in an image intensifier?
_____ a. kVp variations
_____ b. mAs variations
_____ c. video signal variations
_____ d. electrostatic lens variations

87. What determines the penetration energy of an x-ray?
_____ a. the speed of the electron
_____ b. the kVp
_____ c. the type of electron/electron interaction
_____ d. all of the above

88. Which of the following is removed by filtration of the primary beam?
_____ a. long wavelength, high-frequency radiations
_____ b. short wavelength, high-frequency radiations
_____ c. short wavelength, low-frequency radiations
_____ d. long wavelength, low-frequency radiations

89. What is beam harding?
____ a. increasing the peak value
____ b. increasing the percentage of high energy photons
____ c. increasing the percentage of low energy photons
____ d. shifting the modal point of the graph to the left

90. Generally, as the speed of a screen goes down, what happens to the resolution?
____ a. it goes up
____ b. it goes down
____ c. it depends on the type of backing

91. Which of the following affects the speed of an intensifying screen?
____ a. crystal size
____ b. phosphor layer thickness
____ c. phosphor type of screen
____ d. all of the above

92. Which statement is *not* correct about adding antihalation dyes to mammography film?
____ a. The dyes increase speed.
____ b. They reduce the density from screen light.
____ c. They reduce the lateral spread of phosphor light.
____ d. They increase detail

93. Which element has the highest k-shell binding energy?
____ a. W
____ b. Ga
____ c. La
____ d. Y

94. Which of the following will give the greatest radiographic density?
____ a. 50 speed screen
____ b. 100 speed screen
____ c. 200 speed screen
____ d. 300 speed screen

95. Which of the following is true about reciprocal law failure?

I. It occurs frequently in diagnostic imaging.

II. It occurs at very short times.

III. It occurs at very long times.

_____ a. I only

_____ b. I and II only

_____ c. II and III only

_____ d. I, II, and III

96. What is reciprocity law failure?

_____ a. The density of a film goes down when the exposure is very short.

_____ b. The density of a film goes down when the exposure is very long.

_____ c. The density of a film goes up as the exposure is shortened.

_____ d. both a and b

97. Which of the following is the formula for Optical Density (OD)?

_____ a. $\log (10) I_o/I_t$

_____ b. $\log (10) I_t/I_o$

_____ c. $\log (nat) I_o/I_t$

_____ d. $\log (nat) I_t/I_o$

98. Why are some heavy metal filters such as holmium and gadolinium used?

_____ a. to absorb all energy levels except those matched to a contrast media

_____ b. to remove only high energy photons

_____ c. to remove more of the low energy photons

_____ d. to remove the middle range photons

99. What is the best means of preventing developer chemical oxidation?

_____ a. Use replenisher holding tanks that are as large as possible.

_____ b. Store chemicals at recommended temperatures.

     c. Use mixed chemicals within 10–14 days.

     d. Use a floating lid in the developer tank.

100. Which of the following are appropriate uses of average gradient?

     I. a comparison of the published average gradient form films from a specific manufacturer.

     II. as a relative measure of contrast

     III. to compare the contrast of different film-screen combinations

     a. I and II only

     b. I and III only

     c. II and III only

     d. I, II, and III

101. Which of the following film types will have the highest average gradient?

     a. radiation therapy port film

     b. mammogram

     c. chest x-ray

     d. CT scan

102. An exposure of 5 mr shows a density of 0.8 on a radiograph. What density would be shown by 10 mR?

     a. 0.9

     b. 1.1

     c. 1.6

     d. 3.2

103. Which of the following is (are) true about quantum mottle?

     a. Quantum mottle increases with increased film speed.

     b. Quantum mottle increases with increased kVp.

     c. Quantum mottle has the greatest effect on the perceptibility of low-contrast structures.

     d. all of the above

104. Which of the following is (are) true regarding latent image fading?

_____ a. Fading occurs if mammographic images are not processed within one hour.

_____ b. Fading occurs if the sensitometric strip is not processed soon after exposure.

_____ c. Fading occurs on the contrast scale of the image.

_____ d. all of the above

105. Which of the following are reasonable exceptions for latent image fading after 48 hours?

_____ a. Optical density decreases by 0.3.

_____ b. Film speed loss will be 20%.

_____ c. Contrast loss will be 5%.

_____ d. all of the above

106. Which of the following is (are) true about reciprocity law failure?

_____ a. It can be high or low intensity.

_____ b. It occurs at very short and very long exposure times.

_____ c. It produces little change in film contrast.

_____ d. all of the above

107. What term describes the misrepresentation of true image size or shape?

_____ a. crossover blur

_____ b. parallax blur

_____ c. absorption unsharpness

_____ d. distortion

108. What increase in film density could be expected from a 2° F increase in developer temperature?

_____ a. 5%

_____ b. 15%

_____ c. 25%

_____ d. 50%

109. Which of the following is a geometric variable?
_____ a. kVp
_____ b. pathology
_____ c. SID
_____ d. processor temp

ANSWERS TO CHAPTER 5
PHYSICAL PRINCIPLES QUESTIONS

1. **b**   When waves are totally in phase, the resultant composite wave will have increased amplitude (additive of the two); whereas when two waves are totally out of phase (180° out of phase) a wave of reduced amplitude (highest minus lowest) will be produced. Adding waves of various phase relationships will produce a composite wave of greater complexity.

2. **c**   The ripple (maximum drop in voltage expressed as a percentage of V_{max}) of a three-phase, six-pulse generator should be 13.5%; thus 80 – (80 x 13.5% = 10.8) = 69.2 kV.

3. **d**   In a high-frequency unit, the single-phase or three-phase AC voltage waveforms are rectified, and then fed into a DC frequency modulator where the frequency is converted from 60 Hz to the kHz range.

4. **d**   Single-phase units provide the most ripple of 100%, which means that maximum voltage across the tube ranges from 100% to 0%; three-phase, six-pulse units provide 13.5% ripple, meaning that maximum voltage across the tube ranges from 100% to 86.5%; three-phase, twelve-pulse units provide 3.5% ripple, meaning that maximum voltage across the tube ranges from 100% to 96.5%; and high-frequency provide less than 3.5%. Ideally, 0% ripple would exist, which would mean that 100% of the maximum voltage was being delivered across the tube.

5. **d**   Although early anode disks were made entirely of tungsten, today a compound anode disk is used that is made of a base material, usually molybdenum, with a good heat storage density, relatively low density, and a coating layer of tungsten or tungsten alloy (often 90% tungsten and 10% rhenium). The addition of rhenium reduces roughening and cracking of the target surface that can result from thermal stress.

6. **d** Disk size is an important factor, along with disk mass and speed of rotation in determining safe thermal loads; typical anode disks tend to range from 5 cm (2 in.) to 12.5 cm (5 in.) on rotating anodes.

7. **a** If the anode is not tilted, the actual and effective focal spots will be the same size. Thompson uses the term *apparent* focal spot rather than *effective* focal spot.

8. **b** Although an angle is necessary to provide an effective focal spot that is smaller than the actual focal spot, increasing the size of the angle will increase the size of that effective focal spot. The actual focal spot size remains constant.

9. **b** Causes of poor screen-film contact include foreign bodies in cassettes, loose springs and hinges, and twisted or warped frames; and it tends to be more common in larger cassettes.

10. **b** The increased divergence of light caused by the increased space between the film and screen causes an increased divergence of light that appears as a darker area on the film.

11. **b** Fog will increase the overall amount of base + fog in the visible, or manifest, image and decrease contrast. Fog is unwanted since it is a blanket that covers every useful density on the radiograph.

12. **a** Bromide drag, also called bromide flow or directional effect, occurs when the side of the strip with the greatest exposure is fed first into the film processor. Putting the darker end in first causes bromide byproducts to be dragged over the film, which may retard development.

13. **a** When there is a slight contamination of the developer with fixer, the fixer tends to break down the silver bromide crystals, allowing the developer to reduce more unexposed crystals. This increases chemical fog, resulting in an increase in speed and a reduction in contrast.

14. **d** The slope of the $D_{LOG}E$ curve indicates film contrast. A steeper slope indicates higher contrast.

15. **a** Film speed is indicated by the position of $D_{LOG}E$ curve. Faster speed films have their speed points to the left of the film to which they are being compared.

16. **b** Although sources vary somewhat, and base + fog will vary by film and manufacturer; in general, base + fog of an unexposed film should range from 0.1–0.15.

17. **c** Unexposed, processed x-ray film should allow no more than 80% of light to be transmitted through it. A film with an optical density of 0.1 will allow 79% of light to pass through; 0.15 optical density will allow 71% of light to pass through.

18. **d** The average gradient of x-ray films tends to be much larger than 1.0 (which improves subject contrast), and most have average gradients in the range of 2.5–3.5.

19. **a** The slope of the tangent at any point on the characteristic curve defines gradient. There are a number of gradients that can be calculated on the curve, including average gradient and toe gradient.

20. **b** Latitude is the range of exposures over which the x-ray film responds with densities in the diagnostically useful range. A film with a wider range of exposures is said to have greater, or wider, latitude.

21. **d** The level of portion or shoulder of the $D_{LOG}E$ curve is the D_{max}, or maximum density.

22. **d** Improper spectral matching (using a film that does not match the spectral characteristics of the screen) can influence density, contrast, and latitude, as well as patient dose.

23. **b** In mammography, base + fog is allowed to vary within 0.03 of the control value. In general radiography, base + fog is usually allowed to vary with 0.05 of the control value.

24. **c** The higher the temperature, the shorter the life of the chemicals. Above 100° F, chemicals might only last one month; at 70° F, their life is about 12 months.

25. **c** Average gradient is the average of all gradient points on a $D_{LOG}E$ curve that exist between 0.25 and 2.0.

26. **d** Density difference (DD) or contrast is calculated by the difference between the step closest to 2.2 but not below 2.0 and the step closest to but not below 0.45. Thus, in this case one would subtract step 13 from step 9.

27. **d** **Advantages of Molybdenum**
   a. produces more low energy
   b. resultant image has higher contrast
   c. produces x-ray energies

   Disadvantages
   a. less x-ray photon output photons due to lower atomic number
   b. increased mAs requiring radiographic contrast to maintain film density
   c. increases dose to the patient required for breast imaging.

28. **b** With a tungsten target at less than 70 kVp, about 100% of the beam will be bremsstrahlung; at 80 kVp, about 90%, at 150 kVp, about 70%.

29. **b** Changing the "Z" number of the target material affects both the bremsstrahlung radiation production and the characteristic production. If the "Z" number increases, there will be more high energy photons produced as well as a higher characteristic line.

30. **c** Changing mAs will change only the amplitude in both the bremsstrahlung and characteristic areas of the spectrum; energy will be unaffected.

31. **d** Changing the kVp lowers the peak energy, increases the number of lower energy photons produced, and reduces the number of characteristic photons produced.

32. **e** Reducing the filtration increases the number of low energy photons in the beam but does not change the peak energy or the characteristic radiation production.

33. **e** Single-phase radiation production has lower average energy, fewer overall photon production, and fewer characteristic production than three-phase production.

34. **a** When compared with single-phase, three-phase shows about a 12% increase in the number of x-rays; high frequency shows an increase of about 16% over single-phase.

35. **d** In the dryer system in an automatic processor, the tubes used have a slit for air to exit, a temperature of about 120° F is commonly used, and the duct to the outside should be as straight as possible to maintain efficiency.

36. **a** Since crossover racks are positioned partly in solution and partly in air, there is an increased potential for chemical deposits to form on them. This necessitates additional cleaning of these racks.

37. **d** The detection rack or feed rack is the first set of rollers the film comes into contact with. They begin a process that will activate the micro-switch controlling the replenishment system. These are also called entrance rollers.

38. **b** Although unexposed silver halide crystals are mostly unaffected by the developer, there is a small number that can be affected. This results in chemical fog.

39. **a** Enamel, hard-glazed earthenware, polyethylene, polypropylene, glass, hard rubber, and ANSI Type 316 stainless steel with 2–3% molybdenum are considered to be corrosion-resistant materials for the purposes of mixing and storing processor chemistry. Reactive materials such as tin, copper, zinc, aluminum or galvanized iron should never used.

40. **b** The correct order of the assemblies in an automatic processor is entrance roller, racks, turnarounds, crossovers, squeegees, dryer. The number of assemblies and specific designs may vary but the basic plan is the same.

41. **c** The recirculation system uniformly mixes the processing and replenisher solutions, maintains the proper temperature and chemical activity, and keeps thoroughly mixed and agitated solutions in constant contact with the films. The transport systems moves the film through the processor, the water washes films and stabilizes processing temperatures, and replenishment keeps chemicals in their proper portions.

42. **b** Water used for radiographic processing must not necessarily be drinkable; however, if undrinkable water is used, its suitability must be assessed. Excessively hard water and water containing dissolved sulfides may not be suitable.

43. **d** Metallic replacement chemically replaces the silver in solution with another metal, usually iron or steel wool. Electrolytic recovery uses an anode and cathode, and chemical precipitation is a commercial method that adds various compounds to the fixer bath. Reverse osmosis and ion exchange are methods of recovering silver usually used in photo finishing operations.

44. **b** The size of the focal spot as quoted by the manufacturer of equipment is called the nominal focal spot. This is not the same as the measured focal spot.

45. **b** Bromide and gelatin deposits known as reaction particles form on the surface of the film. A large amount of them may cause the developing solution to be unable to react with the exposed silver bromide crystals, resulting in underdevelopment. Agitation is designed to shake these particles loose from the film.

46. **d** The size of the effective focal spot depends on the actual focal spot size and the target angles. The size of the effective focal spot will decrease with smaller actual focal spot sizes and smaller target angles. Focal spot size is also affected by kVp and mA, which can cause focal spot "blooming."

47. **a** Resolution is a geometric image factor, and is expressed in line pairs per millimeter. Although kVp might influence the visibility of detail, it does not directly affect detail. Screen speed and screen-film contact, focal spot size, OID, and SID all affect resolution.

48. **b** Spectral matching is producing equal wavelengths of light; it usually refers to suiting the wavelength of light generated to that of the imaging system. Thus, for film-screen combinations, it involves assuring that the light generated by the screens is the same type of light that the film is most sensitive to.

49. **a** Radiographic contrast is the difference between densities and is a photographic property of the image. It is generally divided into two categories: film and subject. Film, screens, subject (e.g., pathology or tissue composition), development, and kVp are all primary factors in radiographic contrast. Focal spot size will affect the image geometrically.

50. **d** mR/mAs is calculated simply by dividing the exposure in mR by the mAs setting chosen. Thus, here $60 \div 20 = 3$.

51. **b** In mammography, too short of an exposure time may cause grid artifacts, too long of an exposure time may cause reciprocity law failure, and exposure times can vary greatly for breast compressed to the same size due to variations in tissue makeup.

52. **d** In mammography, backup times may be reached due to the inability of the set kVp to penetrate the breast, AECs can be designed to compensate for reciprocity law failure during long exposures, and many new machines have circuits that adjust to the kVp to a higher level by sensing the exposure in the first 100 milliseconds.

53. **b** The cathode end of the tube is place directly over the chest wall side of the image to take advantage of the prominent heel effect of the anode; due to the line-focus principle, resolution is decreased at the chest wall; and the beam is placed off-center to provide a smaller focal spot at the chest wall, as well as allowing the vertical central ray to enter straight in at the chest wall.

54. **a** The advantages of rhodium over molybdenum is that it provides slightly higher kVs, which allow for reductions in exposure times. However, the higher kVp may not be appropriate for smaller breasts.

55. **b** Regulations specify that HVL shall not be less than 0.30 mm Al eq at 30 kVp, the operating capability of mammography equipment. Too high of an HVL (e.g., more than 0.40 mm) will decrease radiographic image contrast.

56. **c** Bias focusing is a process where one filament wire is used for both large and small focal spots and a negative voltage is applied to reduce the size of the electron stream, creating a smaller focal spot.

57. **b** Gamma is a measure of steepness of the $D_{LOG}E$ curve along the straight-line portion, and is often used in industrial and cine radiography and photography. Average gradient is the average of the gradient points that exist between the densities of 0.25 and 2.00, and is commonly used in diagnostic radiography. Toe gradient (between 0.25 and 1.0), middle gradient (between 1.0 and 2.0) and upper gradient (between 2.0 and 2.5) are not widely used.

58. **d** Average gradient is calculated by dividing (D2-D1), which is always 1.75, by (E2-E1), giving in this case, 2.92.

59. **b** In film 1, average gradient is calculated by dividing 1.75 by (E2-E1) (0.7), which gives 2.5. In film 2, average gradient is calculated by dividing 1.75 by 0.9, which gives 1.9. The higher the average gradient, the greater the exaggeration of subject contrast will be; thus film 1 will exaggerate subject contrast more than film 2.

60. **b** Hydroquinone is slow working and is easily oxidized, and thus, is considered to be a weaker developing agent than phenidone. It affects black tones primarily, controls the shoulder of the H&D curve (D_{max}), and thus, is a primary controller of contrast.

61. **d** Phenidone is fast working and plateaus after a time. It controls the grays of the image, influencing the toe of the $D_{LOG}E$ curve, controls the D_{min}, and is the primary controller of film sensitivity or speed.

62. **b** Comparisons between films are only useful if those comparisons are made with the exact type of light used to expose the film (the spectral matching between film and screen). However, for normal quality control purposes, the type of light in the sensitometer does not matter.

63. **a** A film with an average gradient of 1 will not affect subject contrast; less than 1 decreases subject contrast; and more than 1 exaggerates subject contrast. Image size and film-screen contact are geometric factors and are unaffected by a photographic property such as average gradient.

64. **c** Increasing the time or temperature of development will increase average gradient, increasing film contrast; increase film speed; and increase fog, which decreases film contrast.

65. **a** Average gradient and speed are expressed numerically; latitude is not. However, in general, the latitude of a film varies inversely with film contrast.

66. **b** Silver halide will normally absorb light in the ultraviolet, violet, and blue regions of the spectrum. Adding a dye to help it better absorb light in the green spectrum makes it an orthochromatic film; adding a dye that helps it absorb light in the red spectrum, it is called panchromatic film.

67. **b** An increase of 0.3 in log relative exposure represents a doubling of the relative exposure; thus 0.3 = 2x relative exposure; 0.6 = 4x relative exposure, and so on.

68. **b** A doubling of the relative exposure is represented logarithmically by an increase of 0.3; thus a 200 speed film would be represented in the example by 2.3; a 400 speed by 2.6, and so on.

69. **b** If 0.1% of the developer tank's capacity contains fixer, it can become contaminated; thus, for a one gallon (4000 ml) tank, as little as 4 ml of fixer could contaminate the tank.

70. **a** If the processor chemicals were depleted, it would be more gradual and occur at times other than at 4 PM. If the unit was improperly attached to the power source, variations in the output would be noticeable but not just at one time of the day.

71. **b** Although film can resolve up to 100 lp/mm, screens are typically a "weak link" in the imaging chain in that most can only resolve up to about 10 lp/mm. In general, the slower the screen, the greater is resolving power.

72. **b** Films with a high average gradient will tend to have high contrast and speed; also, in general, latitude of a film varies inversely with film contrast.

73. **c** Solarization is the term for the region of reversal once the $D_{LOG}E$ curve passes D_{max}. Theory suggests that this is due to a recombination of silver and bromide; this process should not occur with radiographic films processed in automatic processors.

74. **a** Greater SIDs decrease magnification and also provide a reduced patient exposure, but since increased technical factors must be selected to compensate for the increase in distance, tube loading may increase.

75. **b** Single-emulsion films tend to have slower speeds (and thus a decreased density at the same technical factors), lower contrast, wider latitude, and better recorded detail.

76. **d** Light reflected back at the film (base-air interface) will cause the formation of a diffuse "halo" (the process of halation), which will cause some loss of recorded detail. This problem is solved by adding an antihalation layer to single-emulsion film, which can be recognized as the glossy side of the film.

77. **c** Duplication film is designed so that longer exposure times result in less density, thus their $D_{LOG}E$ curves appear to be the opposite of radiographic films, beginning with high densities on the left side of the curve and terminating with low densities.

78. **c** Hydroquinone, metol, and phenidone are the three most common reducing agents (developers). The function of the reducing agents in the developer is to donate electrons to the exposed silver bromide crystals and reduce them to elemental silver. Elemental silver makes up the black portion of the radiograph.

79. **b** In order for the reducing (development) to take place, the proper pH must be present. The developer is slightly basic or alkaline.

80. **a** The function of the fixer is to stop development, remove unexposed crystals, and fix the image for archival storage. In order to stop the development, the fixer is very acidic.

81. **a** Phenidone is responsible for development of the gray tones on a radiograph and works faster than hydroquinone, which is the other reducer found in most developers.

82. **d** Hydroquinone is the principal reducing agent in developer. It is responsible for development of the black tones on a radiograph and works slower than phenidone, which is the other reducer usually found in developers.

83. **c** Metal salt ions build up in the developer. These speed up the oxidation of hydroquinone and reduce the effectiveness of the developer. Chelates sequester ions and prevent them from attacking the developer.

84. **a** The fixer must be acidotic and acetate is added to the solution to help maintain the pH.

85. **a** Optical Density (OD) is based on the log value of the percentage of light that does not pass through a film. The formula is $OD = \text{Log}(10)\ I_o/I_t$. If $I_o = I_t$, then $\text{Log}(10)$ of $1 = 0.00$.

86. **d** Fluoroscopic brightness is controlled be varying the mA, the kVp, or the video signal. If only variation of mAs and kVp are used, it is sometimes called automatic dose rate control. When video signal is varied, it is called automatic gain control. The sensitivity of the camera can also be controlled, which is called automatic brightness control.

87. **d** The potential difference of the x-ray tube is measured in kVp and controls the speed of the electrons as they hit the anode. The speed of the electrons impacts the types of interactions (brems at different energies and characteristics).

88. **d** Low "Z" number materials, such as aluminum, are used for filters as they tend to absorb mostly low energy, low frequency, long wavelength radiation.

89. **b** Beam harding is the process of removing low energy photons, leaving only the higher energy ones in the beam. Harding the beam reduces patient dose and scatter formation.

90. **a** Generally, anything that increases the speed of a screen (with the exception of going from CaWO4 to rare earth) will decrease detail formation. Increasing the size of the phosphors, increasing the thickness of the phosphor layer, removing the antihalation dyes, and adding a reflective backing increase speed.

91. **d** Increasing the size of the phosphors, increasing the thickness of the phosphor layer, removing the anti-halation dyes, and adding a reflective backing increase speed and reduce recorded detail. Going from CaWO4 to rare earth increases speed without loss of detail.

92. **a** Antihalation dye is a coating added to any single-sided film to reduce reflection of screen light transmitted through the emulsion and base.

93. **a** The binding energy of the k-shell electron determines the probability of a photoelectric interaction and is important in screen technology as well as contrast media. The k-shell binding energy of Tungsten (W) is approximately 70 keV, Gadolinium (Ga) is 64 keV, Lanthanum (La) is 57 keV, and Yttrium (Y) is 39.

94. **d** The speed of a screen is relative and linear. The higher the number, the faster the speed. Doubling the number, doubles the speed.

95. **c** Reciprocity law failure is the reduction in density at very long and very short exposure times. It is almost never seen with short times in diagnostic radiology, but is occasionally seen with the long exposure times in mammography.

96. **d** Reciprocity Law states that when an exposure is very long (such as in mammography) or very short (not

usually seen in diagnostic radiology) the density may be reduced below that expected from given mAs.

97. a Optical Density (OD) is based on the log value of the percent of light that does not pass through a film. The formula being OD = Log(10) Io/It.

98. a Filters such as holmium have a k-edge slightly above the k-edge of iodine and leave energy levels that have a much higher probability of having a photoelectric interaction with the iodine. This makes the contrast media more visible on the radiograph.

99. d Typically, a replenisher holding tank large enough to hold a week's worth of chemicals should be used. Although storing chemicals at recommended temperatures and using mixed chemicals within 10 to 14 days are both good means of preventing oxidation, the best prevention is to use a floating lid in the developer tank.

100. a Average gradient can be used to compare the published average gradient for films from a specific manufacturer or as a relative measure of contrast; it should not be used to compare the contrast of different film-screen combinations.

101. a Radiation therapy port films will have an average gradient of about 5.7; mammogram, about 3.3; general purpose x-ray, about 2.8; chest x-ray, about 2.2; CT and MR, about 1.9-2.5.

102. b A change of 0.3 is roughly a doubling; thus if 5 mR is recorded as 0.8, then 10 mR should show a density of 1.1.

103. d Quantum mottle is the effect of using a limited number of x-ray quanta to form the image. It increases with increased film speed and kVp; and has the greatest effect on the perceptibility of low-contrast structures such as cysts or soft tissue lesions.

104. b Latent image fading should not be significant as long as mammographic images are processed by the end of the day. It may, however, have a significant effect on the sensitometric strip. It causes little change in contrast scale.

105. **d** Haus and Jaskulski give a loss of 0.27 for optical density, percent speed loss of 23%, and contrast loss of 5% as an example of latent image fading.

106. **d** Reciprocity law failure can be high or low intensity, occurring at very short and very long exposure times. It typically requires additional exposure, and may be a problem in mammography, where long exposure times are used. It produces little change in film contrast.

107. **d** Misrepresentation of true size (magnification) or shape are both forms of distortion.

108. **a** 2° increase in temperature would increase film density by about 15%.

109. **c** Of all the variables listed, the one that is most clearly a geometric variable is SID or source-to-image receptor distance.

MULTIPLE-CHOICE QUESTIONS

1. How many wires per inch should the copper wire mesh used to test screen-film contact contain?
   ____ a. 10
   ____ b. 20
   ____ c. 40
   ____ d. 80

2. There is no need to warm up the densitometer prior to reading QC strips.
   ____ a. true
   ____ b. false

3. What are the typical spoke angles used for a star test pattern?
   ____ a. 0.5 to 2.0°
   ____ b. 1.0 to 2.0°
   ____ c. 2.0 to 4.0°
   ____ d. 2.0 to 5.0°

4. What term describes the intensity of light falling on a surface from other sources?
   ____ a. illuminance
   ____ b. luminance
   ____ c. extraneous light
   ____ d. color

5. What is the unit for luminance?
   ____ a. candela (cd/m^2)
   ____ b. lumen/m^2
   ____ c. lux
   ____ d. two of the above

6. What is the maximum readable density with a brightness of 1500 cd/m^2?
   ____ a. OD 0.8
   ____ b. OD 1.8
   ____ c. OD 2.8
   ____ d. OD 3.8

7. No contrast will be lost with ambient lighting of 50 lux.
   ____ a. true
   ____ b. false

8. Which of the following is not a key element in providing the best possible lighting for reading films?
   ____ a. proper luminance
   ____ b. eliminating extraneous light
   ____ c. use of homogeneous light source
   ____ d. increasing ambient light (luminance)

9. How many nit equal 3000 cd/m^2 (candelas)?
   ____ a. 1000   ____ c. 6000
   ____ b. 3000   ____ d. 10000

10. What term describes ambient light + extraneous light?
    ____ a. luminance
    ____ b. illuminance
    ____ c. lux
    ____ d. none of the above

11. What is the typical incremental log exposure provided by simulated light sensitometers?
    ____ a. OD 0.05
    ____ b. OD 0.10
    ____ c. OD 0.15
    ____ d. OD 0.30

12. Which of the following is (are) true about simulated light sensitometers?
    _____ a. Canned air, shaken prior to use, should be used for cleaning.
    _____ b. The area in which it is used should be temperature controlled (59–86° F)
    _____ c. Recalibration should not be necessary.
    _____ d. all of the above

13. Which of the following are types of densitometers?
    _____ a. spot-reading
    _____ b. manual
    _____ c. automatic
    _____ d. all of the above

14. What is the usual setting on a sensitometer for single-emulsion mammography film?
    _____ a. single and green
    _____ b. single and blue
    _____ c. double and green
    _____ d. double and blue

15. Which of the following is (are) true about the apertures of spot-reading densitometers?
    _____ a. Large apertures require less accuracy in positioning.
    _____ b. Large apertures produce a better signal-to-noise ration.
    _____ c. Large apertures provide less reliable results.
    _____ d. all of the above

16. It is mandatory to check the response of radiation detection instruments using an appropriate radiation source?
    _____ a. true
    _____ b. false

17. Which of the following is best used for qualitative, rather then quantitative, low-level radiation exposure measurements?
    _____ a. personnel monitoring device
    _____ b. Geiger-Mueller counter
    _____ c. portable scintillation detector
    _____ d. ionization chamber

18. How many chamber are in the move kVp meters?
    _____ a. 1
    _____ b. 2
    _____ c. 3
    _____ d. 5

19. Which of the following is not normally used for radiation detection in kVp meters?
    _____ a. ion chambers
    _____ b. photo diodes
    _____ c. voltage diodes

20. When using a sensitometer, how often should they be calibrated?
    _____ a. yearly
    _____ b. bi-yearly
    _____ c. monthly
    _____ d. never

21. Which of the following devices uses an optical step-wedge?
    _____ a. densitometer
    _____ b. dosimeter
    _____ c. penetrometer
    _____ d. sensitometer

22. What type of film is used specifically for sensitometry in a general diagnostic department?
    _____ a. the same film most commonly used in the department
    _____ b. the fastest film used in the department
    _____ c. non-screen film, as no screen was used
    _____ d. the most processor sensitive film

23. What is the most appropriate type of sensitometry film to use in a processor where general and mammography film is processed?

    _____ a. the most processor sensitive film
    _____ b. mammography film
    _____ c. the fastest film in the department
    _____ d. the most commonly used film in the department

24. Which type of thermometer should *not* be used in a processor?

    _____ a. mercury type
    _____ b. analog type
    _____ c. electrified
    _____ d. metric

25. What is the temperature range that a processor developer thermometer should have?

    _____ a. 0–150° F
    _____ b. 50–125° F
    _____ c. 90–108° F
    _____ d. 95–100° F

26. Of the following types of thermometers, which type is recommended for use in a processor?

    _____ a. digital
    _____ b. alcohol
    _____ c. mercury
    _____ d. analog

27. What is the acceptable level of accuracy for a developer solution thermometer?

    _____ a. 2° F
    _____ b. 1° F
    _____ c. 0.5° F
    _____ d. 0.3° F

28. What is the typical incremental log exposure difference between steps on a sensitometer?

    _____ a. OD 0.10
    _____ b. OD 0.15
    _____ c. OD 0.25
    _____ d. OD 0.25

29. What type of sensitometer is recommended for processor QC?
    _____ a. single-sided exposure
    _____ b. double-sided exposure
    _____ c. varies depending on situation
    _____ d. none of the above

30. Which of the following is not a requirement for a sensitometer?
    _____ a. blue and green light emissions
    _____ b. single-or double-sided exposures
    _____ c. adjustable light intensity
    _____ d. none of the above

31. A simulated light sensitometer can be used for film speed and contrast evaluations.
    _____ a. true
    _____ b. false

32. When using mammography film for sensitometry, what setting should be used?
    _____ a. green and single
    _____ b. green and double
    _____ c. blue and single
    _____ d. blue and double

33. When using asymmetric near-zero crossover film in sensitometry, what is used to compensate for the different emulsions on either side of the film?
    _____ a. double exposures
    _____ b. spectral mismatching
    _____ c. graduated filters
    _____ d. neutral density filter

34. Which of the following is *not* a type of densitometer?
    _____ a. automatic scanning densitometer
    _____ b. mammographic phantom densitometer
    _____ c. spot reading densitometer
    _____ d. none of the above

35. What aperture diameter is recommended for use on a densitometer?
_____ a. 1 mm
_____ b. 2 mm
_____ c. 3mm
_____ d. none of the above

36. When using a densitometer, how often should it be calibrated?
_____ a. yearly
_____ b. bi-yearly
_____ c. monthly
_____ d. never

37. How accurately should a densitometer be calibrated?
_____ a. ± .01 OD
_____ b. ± .02 OD
_____ c. ± .05 OD
_____ d. ± .10 OD

38. What color light is used in a densitometer?
_____ a. blue
_____ b. green
_____ c. yellow
_____ d. white

ANSWERS TO CHAPTER 6
TEST INSTRUMENTATION QUESTIONS

1. **c** In testing for screen-film contact, a test tool containing at least 40 wires per inch grid density is placed directly on the cassette.

2. **b** The densitometer should be turned on at least 10 to 15 minutes before QC strips are read. Not doing so may produce values outside control limits. Smaller, portable densitometers require less warm-up time.

3. **a** The spoke angles used for the star pattern are typically form 0.5–2.0°, 0.5° for focal spots less than 0.3 mm, 1° for focal spots of 0.3–0.6 mm, 1.5° for 0.6–1.2 mm, and 2° for focal spots above 1.2 mm.

4. **a** The intensity of light falling on a surface from other sources describes illuminance. Luminance is the intensity of light at the surface of the illuminator.

5. **a** The unit for luminance is candela (cd/m^2) or the nit, which are identical measures. Lumen/m^2 or lux are measurements of illuminance.

6. **c** The maximum readable density with a brightness of 1500 cd/m^2 is OD 2.8; with 3000/m^2, it is OD 3.1

7. **b** 50 lux, which is about equivalent to a moonlit night, can remove as much as 30% of the contrast from a film.

8. **d** Proper luminance, eliminating extraneous light, use of a homogeneous light source (luminance uniformity), and minimizing ambient light (luminance) are all key elements in providing the best possible lighting for reading films.

9. **b** 3000 cd/m^2 (candelas) are equal to 3000 nit. They are equivalent units.

10. **d** There is no entity that consists of the combination of ambient light and extraneous light. Ambient light is also known as illuminance, and its unit is lumen/m^2 or lux. Extraneous light is light coming from the viewer outside of the area being examined.

11. **c**   Simulated light sensitometers are devices used to expose x-ray film to different light intensities in a step fashion; each step or incremental log exposure is typically 0.15.

12. **b**   Canned air should be used for cleaning a sensitometer; however, it should not be shaken prior to use. The area should be temperature controlled from 59–86° F, and recalibration may be necessary as the tungsten light source or electro luminescent panel ages.

13. **d**   Types of densitometers include spot-reading (also called manual) and automatic.

14. **a**   There are two settings on most simulated light sensitometers; one is exposure (single or dual), another is color (blue or green). For single-emulsion mammography film, the usual setting is single and green.

15. **b**   Spot-reading densitometers usually provide different size apertures such as 1, 2, and 3 millimeters. The large apertures require greater accuracy in positioning, but provide a better signal-to-noise ratio and more reliable results.

16. **a**   the response of radiation detection instruments shall be checked periodically using an appropriate radiation source; whereas the RSO (radiation safety officer) should be consulted prior to the procurement of survey meters.

17. **b**   Geiger-Mueller counters are very sensitive and useful for the qualitative measurement of low levels of radiation; they tend to over-respond to low levels of radiation. Ionization chambers are less energy-dependent and give a more accurate depiction of exposure; whereas portable scintillation detectors are sensitive to low-level photons such as those emitted from iodine-125.

18. **b**   In most kVp meters, there are either two ion chambers or photo diodes. The amount of filtration differs between the two chambers and, based on the difference in absorption, kVp can be calculated.

19. **c** Both the ion chamber and photo diode are commonly used radiation detection components in kVp meters. Voltage diodes and oscilloscopes are also used for kVp measurement because they are more accurate than ion chambers or photo diodes. However, it takes significantly longer to use them, so they are not commonly used.

20. **a** The Bureau of Radiologic Health recommends that a sensitometer be calibrated monthly, but that recommendations was made in the 1970s. Most sensitometers come with a recommendation to be calibrated yearly.

21. **d** A sensitometer is used to deliver a graduated light exposure to film for use in processor quality control. In order to do that, a light emitting crystal is covered by an optical step-wedge to give the film exposure graduation.

22. **d** When selecting film to be used with a sensitometer, the type most sensitive to processor changes is the most appropriate choice. This allows the QM technologists to detect changes in the processor sooner.

23. **b** Because of the special nature of mammography film, only this type of film should be used in a processor that deals with a mixed set of film types.

24. **a** Mercury is a heavy metal similar to silver and, if a mercury thermometer broke inside a processor, the mercury would interact with and contaminate the chemicals. Unfortunately, because mercury is liquid at room temperature, it would tend to get into the recirculating systems and elsewhere in the processor and continue to contaminate the chemicals for some time.

25. **c** Most processor developer solutions are maintained around 95° F. Also, as the range of the thermometer increases, the accuracy decreases. Based on those two facts, most thermometers have a range of 90–108° F. This makes this specialty thermometer useless for measuring temperatures in the fixer or water.

26. **a** The digital thermometer is recommended because of its ability to measure units as little as one-tenth of a degree, and because they can not contaminate the solution. Analog thermometers are less accurate as digital ones. Any glass type thermometer, such as alcohol and mercury, should not be used because of the possibility of breakage and contamination.

27. **c** A thermometer should be accurate within 0.5° F for use in a processor 0.5° F is equivalent to 0.3° C.

28. **b** In most sensitometers, the log exposure difference between steps is OD 0.15. this gives approximately a 40% difference in density from step to step.

29. **c** Whether a sensitometer is set for single- or double-sided exposure is determined by the type of film being used for sensitometry. If mammography film is used, it is a singe-emulsion film and, therefore, the sensitometer should be set for single-sided exposure. If a general diagnostic film is used, double-sided exposure is preferred.

30. **c** All sensitometers should be able to emit blue or green light as needed. If a sensitometer is capable of giving a double-sided exposure, there needs to be a switch to turn off one side when exposing single-emulsion film. As the main function of the sensitometer is to give consistent exposures, adjusting the light intensity is not advisable. Many sensitometers do have dip switches on the back to set the intensity based on the type of film being use.

31. **b** The light emitted from a sensitometer is different in intensity and distribution compared to that emitted by intensifying screens, and the film reacts differently to the two sources. Therefore, the response from the two sources will differ, making an evaluation based on sensitometry data not appropriate.

32. **a** Best results are obtained from the sensitometry process when the setting best matches the film being used. Mammography film is green sensitive and single-sided emulsion so the settings should be green and single.

33. **a** Certain types of films have a different (asymmetric) type of emulsion on each side. Often with these types of film, no light passes from one side of the emulsion to the other (near-zero crossover). The most common use of these film types is in chest radiography. Because of these characteristics, a neutral density filter is used to achieve a front-to-back light ratio similar to the screens used with this type of film.

34. **b** The spot-reading densitometer is the most commonly used densitometer. It gives a transmission reading that must be manually recorded after the film is manually placed. An automatic scanning densitometer reads all steps on a sensitometric film at one time and prints out processor QC information plus any other desired information.

35. **c** Any aperture can be used with a densitometer but a larger aperture is recommended. As the size of the aperture increases, the precision of the position needs to increase but the signal-to-noise ratio decreases. Therefore, better results are obtained with a larger aperture and accurate positioning.

36. **a** Densitometers should be calibrated at least once a year. In order to do this, use the calibration strip that was returned with the densitometer the last time it was calibrated at the factory. These calibration strips must be traceable to the National Institute of Standards and Technology.

37. **b** A densitometers should be calibrated to OD .02 or 2.5%, whichever is greater.

38. **d** As a densitometer is designed to measure the percentage (in log values) of light transmitted from a typical illuminator, white light is used.

Suggested Readings

Adams, H. G., & Arora, S. (1994). *Total quality in radiology: A guide to implementation.* Boca Raton, FL: Saint Lucie Press.

Adler, A., Carlton, R., & Wold, B. (1992). A comparison of student radiographic reject rates. *Radiologic Technology 64* (1): 26–32.

American College of Radiology Committee on Quality Assurance in Mammography (1999). *Mammography quality control manual.* Reston, VA: Author.

Burns, C. (1995). Achieving darkroom and processing quality control in mammography: A step beyond minimum recommendations. *Seminars in Radiologic Technology 3*(2): 68–85.

Burns, N, & Grove, S. K. (2001). *The practice of nursing research: Conduct, critique & utilization.* Philadelphia: WB Saunders.

Bushberg, J. T., Seibert, J. A., Leidholdt, E. M., et al. (1994). *The essential physics of medial imaging.* Baltimore: Williams and Wilkins.

Bushong, S. (1997). *Radiologic science for technologists: Physics, biology, and protection.* St. Louis: Mosby.

Carlton, R. R., Adler, A., & Burns, B. (2000). *Principles of radiographic imaging: An art and a science.* Albany, NY: Delmar.

Carroll, Q. B. (1998). *Fuch's radiographic exposure, processing & quality control.* Springfield, IL: CC Thomas Publisher.

Chaff, L. F. (1994). *Safety guide for health care institutions.* Chicago: American Hospital Publishing, Inc.

Claflin, N. (1998). *NAHQ guide to quality management.* Glenview, IL: National Association for Healthcare Quality.

Correctec. (1998). *Quality management advanced examination.* (Computer Software) Athens, GA: Author.

Curry, T. S., Dowdey, J. E., & Murry, R. C. (1990). *Christensen's physics of diagnostic radiology.* Philadelphia, PA: Lippincott, Williams & Wilkins.

Dowd, S. B., & Tilson, E. (1996). The benefits of using CQI/TQM data. *Radiologic Technology 67*(6): 533–537.

Dowd, S. B., & Tilson, E. (1998). *Quality management examination review.* (Computer Software) Edwardsville, KS: Educational Software Concepts.

Eastman Kodak. (undated). *The fundamentals of radiography* (12th ed.). Rochester, NY: Author.

Frank, E. (1995). The design and application of the mammography x-ray generator and x-ray tube. *Seminars in Radiologic Technology 3*(2): 56–87.

Giesberg, D. J. (1997). Film viewing condition in mammography. *Radiologic Technology 68*: 429–431.

Haus, A. G., & Jaskulski, S. M. (1997). *The basics of film processing in medical imaging.* Madison, WI: Medial Physics Publishing.

Hiss, S. S. (1997). *Introduction to health care delivery and radiology administration.* Philadelphia: WB Saunders.

Hiss, S. S. (1993). *Understanding radiography* (3rd ed.). Springfield, IL: CC Thomas Publisher.

Jenkins, D. (1980). *Radiographic photography and imaging processes.* Baltimore: University Park Press.

Lam, R., & Golden, L. (1996). *Continuous quality improvement for hospital radiology services. Part 1: Understanding the JCAHO process.* Albuquerque, NM: American Society of Radiologic Technologists.

Lam, R., & Golden, L. (1996). *Continuous quality improvement for hospital radiology services. Part 2: Implementing a successful CQI program.* Albuquerque, NM: American Society of Radiologic Technologist. (Homestudy).

Levin, J. (1983). *Elementary statistics for social research* (3rd ed.). New York: Harper and Row.

McKinney, W. E. J. (1988). *Radiographic processing and quality control.* Philadelphia: JB Lippincott.

McKinney, W. E. J. (1995). *Radiographic processing and quality control.* Los Angeles, CA: Academy Medical Systems.

McKinney, W. E. J. (1997). Analyzing trend charts. *Radiologic Technology 68*(4): 343–344.

McLaughlin, C. P., & Kaluzny, A. D. (1999). *Continuous quality improvement in health care: Theory implementation, and applications.* Gaithersburg, MD: Aspen.

National Council on Radiation Protection and Measurements. (1988). *Report 99: Quality assurance for diagnostic imaging equipment.* Bethesda, MD: Author.

National Council on Radiation Protection and Measurements. (1989). *Report 102: Medical x-ray, electron beam and gamma-ray protection for energies up to 50 MeV (Equipment design, performance and use).* Bethesda, MD: Author.

National Council on Radiation Protection and measurements. (1998). *Report 105: Radiation protection for medical and allied health personnel.* Bethesda, MD: Author.

NEMA Standards Publication No. XR-5-1984. (1984). *Measurement of dimensions and properties of focal spots of diagnostic x-ray tubes.* Washington, DC: Author.

Obergfell, A. M. (1995). *Law & ethics in diagnostic imaging & therapeutic radiology: With risk management and safety applications.* Philadelphia: WB Saunders.

Papp, J. (1998). *Quality management in the imaging sciences.* St. Louis: Mosby.

Thompson, M. A., Hattaway, M. P., Hall, J. D., & Dowd, S. B. (1994). *Principles of imaging science and protection.* Philadelphia: WB Saunders.

Timmereck, T. C. (1997). *Health services cyclopedic dictionary: A compendium of health-care and public health terminology.* Sudbury, MA: Jones and Bartlett.

Tortorici, M. (1992). *Concepts in medical radiographic imaging: Circuitry, exposure & quality control.* Philadelphia: WB Saunders Company.

Towsley, D. (undated). *Customer service: A commitment to quality.* Albuquerque, NM: American Society of Radiologic Technologists. (Homestudy).

U.S. Government. (1994). *OSHA Guideline CPL 2-2.60 – Exposure control plan for OSHA personnel with occupational exposure to bloodborne pathogens.* Washington, DC: United States Government Printing Office.

U.S. Government. (2000). *Code of federal regulations, Title 21, food & drugs, Pt. 1300-end.* Washington, DC: United States Government Printing Office.

Post-test

MULTIPLE-CHOICE QUESTIONS

1. The production of this type of radiation results in very specific energies characterized by the differences between electron binding energies of the target material.
   - ____ a. Bremsstrahlung
   - ____ b. photoelectric
   - ____ c. characteristic
   - ____ d. gamma

2. The atomic number of the target affects both the quantity and quality of the x-rays produced. As the atomic number of the target ____, the efficiency of the production of Bremsstrahlung radiation ____.
   - ____ a. increases, increases
   - ____ b. increases, decreases
   - ____ c. decreases, decreases
   - ____ d. decreases, increases

3. Material that emits light in response to outside stimulation is said to:
   - ____ a. luminesce
   - ____ b. fluoresce
   - ____ c. phosphoresce
   - ____ d. lag

4. A collection of negatively charged electrons forming a small cloud around the filament is termed:
   - ____ a. electron wall
   - ____ b. space effect
   - ____ c. electron emission
   - ____ d. space charge

5. Radiation produced by the interaction of high-speed electrons and metal surfaces other than the focal track of the anode is termed:
   ___ a. scatter radiation
   ___ b. off-focus radiation
   ___ c. secondary radiation
   ___ d. both a and b

6. This component of an intensifying screen is largely composed of cellulose mixed with other polymers. It provides a surface that can be cleaned.
   ___ a. base layer
   ___ b. reflective layer
   ___ c. phosphor layer
   ___ d. protective layer

7. The ability of light emitted by the phosphor of an intensifying screen to escape from the screen and expose the film is termed the:
   ___ a. screen efficiency
   ___ b. intensification factor
   ___ c. conversion efficiency
   ___ d. phosphor factor

8. What results from statistical fluctuation in the number of x-ray photons absorbed by the intensifying screens to form the light image recorded on film?
   ___ a. noise
   ___ b. quantum mottle
   ___ c. distortion
   ___ d. more than one but not all of the above

9. The two most important ingredients of a photographic emulsion are:
   ___ a. gelatin and bromide
   ___ b. silver halide and gelatin
   ___ c. bromide and silver halide
   ___ d. none of the above

10. For radiographic film the sensitivity speck is usually located on the surface of the:
   ___ a. gelatin
   ___ b. bromide crystals
   ___ c. silver halide crystals
   ___ d. none of the above

11. Subjecting radiographs to a combination of low humidity, high temperatures, and other stress such as bending may result in:
    _____ a. cracking artifacts
    _____ b. static artifacts
    _____ c. slap lines
    _____ d. skivings

12. This agent in the high-temperature alkaline developer solution hardens the film to prevent excessive swelling of the gelatin and damage to the film.
    _____ a. sodium sulfite
    _____ b. potassium alum
    _____ c. ammonium thiosulfate
    _____ d. glutaraldehyde

13. The consequences of incomplete fixing become manifest after the image has been stored for some time. These include:
    _____ a. brown films
    _____ b. slap lines
    _____ c. spots of nonuniform density
    _____ d. all of the above

14. This term is defined as the ratio of the mass of a body to the mass of an equal volume of water at a specified temperature.
    _____ a. fluence
    _____ b. granularity
    _____ c. halation
    _____ d. specific gravity

15. The pH measurement indicates the:
    _____ a. acidity of a solution at a specified temperature
    _____ b. alkalinity of a solution at a specified temperature
    _____ c. both a and b
    _____ d. none of the above

16. Starter solution mainly adds _____ ions to the developer.
    _____ a. bromide
    _____ b. antifog
    _____ c. sulfate
    _____ d. sulfide

17. The advantages of room light processing areas include:
   ____ a. more flexibility in processing certain special-ty films
   ____ b. lower investment in equipment
   ____ c. effective use of people
   ____ d. more than one but not all of the above

18. The purpose of the ____ is to help avoid corrosion to the sensitive electronic components of the processor.
   ____ a. dryer exhaust
   ____ b. processor ventilation
   ____ c. both a and b
   ____ d. none of the above

19. A floating lid should always be used on top of the developer replenisher to reduce evaporation and:
   ____ a. chemical oxidation
   ____ b. environmental hazards
   ____ c. accidental spillage
   ____ d. unnecessary replenishment

20. The exposure time accuracy should be checked:
   ____ a. annually
   ____ b. semiannually
   ____ c. monthly
   ____ d. bimonthly

21. A manual spin top test on a single-phase radiographic room only demonstrates half the expected number of dots. What conclusion do you draw from this test?
   ____ a. faulty AEC
   ____ b. faulty rectification
   ____ c. faulty timer
   ____ d. more than one but not all of the above

22. The recommended frequency for testing light field/beam alignment is:
   ____ a. annually
   ____ b. semiannually
   ____ c. monthly
   ____ d. weekly

23. When testing light field/beam alignment, at a 48-inch SID, the light represented light field should be within ±:

_____ a. .48 inches
_____ b. .96 inches
_____ c. 1.44 inches
_____ d. none of the above

24. When testing kilovoltage accuracy, the kilovoltage should be within ±:

_____ a. 6 kVp
_____ b. 5 kVp
_____ c. 4 kVp
_____ d. 2 kVp

25. A reciprocity test for mAs should result in a value of ±:

_____ a. 2%
_____ b. 5%
_____ c. 10%
_____ d. none of the above

26. Which of the following values would be acceptable when testing a three-phase generator for radiation output? The kVp used when performing the test was 80.

_____ a. 5.12 mR/mAs
_____ b. 8.96 mR/mAs
_____ c. 13.44 mR/mAs
_____ d. 20.48 mR/mAs

27. A test for exposure linearity should be performed:

_____ a. annually
_____ b. semiannually
_____ c. monthly
_____ d. weekly

28. The following data are obtained to evaluate exposure linearity. Do the values indicate that the mAs stations are in need of calibration?

| 200 ms | 50 mA | 45 mR |
| 200 ms | 100 mA | 84 mR |

_____ a. yes
_____ b. no

29. This procedure is designed to confirm that the installed tube filtration is acceptable in minimizing exposure to the patient.
_____ a. exposure reproducibility
_____ b. exposure dose linearity
_____ c. half-value layer
_____ d. more than one but not all of the above

30. The three steps necessary for an acceptable QC program are:
_____ a. routine performance monitoring, record keeping, and maintenance
_____ b. acceptance testing, routine performance monitoring, and maintenance
_____ c. acceptance testing, routine performance monitoring, and record keeping
_____ d. routine performance monitoring, analysis, and record keeping

31. The grid uniformity test should insure that the grid:
_____ a. is not producing artifacts
_____ b. is appropriate for portable radiography
_____ c. is aligned with the tabletop and x-ray beam
_____ d. none of the above

32. When testing a grid for alignment, the _____ hole should have the highest optical density with _____ densities to either side.
_____ a. center, increasing
_____ b. center, decreasing
_____ c. aligned, increasing
_____ d. aligned, decreasing

33. Tomographic equipment should be tested to confirm section level is accurate:
_____ a. annually
_____ b. semiannually
_____ c. monthly
_____ d. weekly

34. At a 72-inch SID, which of the following values is acceptable when testing the collimator?
_____ a. 2.8 inches _____ c. 1.5 inches
_____ b. 2 inches _____ d. 1.2 inches

35. The testing frequency for fluoroscopic beam limitation is:
_____ a. annually
_____ b. semiannually
_____ c. monthly
_____ d. weekly

36. High-contrast fluoroscopic resolution testing is designed to verify that the resolution of the imaging system is within acceptable limits. What is an acceptable limit when testing in the 6-inch mode?
_____ a. 40 mesh/inch at the center of the image and 30 mesh/inch at the edge
_____ b. 50 mesh/inch at the center of the image and 30 mesh/inch at the edge
_____ c. 50 mesh/inch at the center of the image and 35 mesh/inch at the edge
_____ d. 40 mesh/inch at the center of the image and 35 mesh/inch at the edge

37. How often should the processor crossover racks be cleaned?
_____ a. daily
_____ b. weekly
_____ c. biweekly
_____ d. monthly

38. The film transport time should not exceed ____% of the recommended manufacturer's processing time.
_____ a. 1 _____ c. 3
_____ b. 2 _____ d. 4

39. The test for illuminator uniformity should be performed:
_____ a. weekly
_____ b. monthly
_____ c. semiannually
_____ d. annually

40. For general radiography, the acceptable parameters for contrast index are:
_____ a. ±0.10
_____ b. ±0.15
_____ c. ±0.5
_____ d. none of the above are acceptable

41. When storing unexposed radiographic film, the relative humidity should be between:

_____ a. 20 to 30%

_____ b. 30 to 50%

_____ c. 40 to 60%

_____ d. more than one but not all of the above

42. The manufacturer's recommended developer temperature for your processor is 92°F. Which of the following values is an acceptable temperature?

_____ a. 98°F

_____ b. 97°F

_____ c. 87°F

_____ d. more than one but not all of the above

43. When using the wire-mesh tool to check for screen-film contact, the technologist should view the results from a distance of _____ away from the viewbox.

_____ a. 2 to 3 m

_____ b. 3 to 4 m

_____ c. 4 to 5 m

_____ d. none of the above

44. For general radiography, the acceptable repeat rate should be less than:

_____ a. 10%

_____ b. 7%

_____ c. 5%

_____ d. 4%

45. Which of the following is not needed to perform processor QC monitoring?

_____ a. sensitometer

_____ b. step wedge

_____ c. densitometer

_____ d. thermometer

46. What is the proper corrective action when the speed index is too high?

_____ a. check developer thermostat setting

_____ b. check replenishment rates

_____ c. check processor overflow drain

_____ d. add developer starter solution

47. The ACR suggests that sensitometers be recalibrated every:
    ____ a. year
    ____ b. 18 months
    ____ c. 2 years
    ____ d. there is no recommendation for periodic recalibration of sensitometers

48. Lead protective devices should be tested for cracks and other defects:
    ____ a. weekly
    ____ b. monthly
    ____ c. semiannually
    ____ d. annually

49. A safelight test has resulted in an unacceptable level of film density. What might cause this result?
    ____ a. a crack in the filter
    ____ b. wrong wattage of bulb in the safelight
    ____ c. improper processing
    ____ d. more than one but not all of the above

50. The mid-range density of the processor control strip reflects the ____ index.
    ____ a. speed
    ____ b. contrast
    ____ c. density
    ____ d. more than one but not all of the above

51. For mammography, a repeat analysis should be performed:
    ____ a. monthly
    ____ b. quarterly
    ____ c. semiannually
    ____ d. annually

52. The digital thermometer used to measure the developer temperature must be accurate to at least ±:
    ____ a. 0.03°F
    ____ b. 0.3°F
    ____ c. 0.05°F
    ____ d. 0.5°F

53. The sensitometer used for mammography QC programs should have _____ steps.
___ a. 21
___ b. 18
___ c. 15
___ d. 10

54. To minimize artifacts on mammography images, dark-room overhead air vents and safelights should be wiped or vacuumed:
___ a. daily
___ b. weekly
___ c. monthly
___ d. quarterly

55. When establishing processor QC operating levels, the mid-density is determined by selecting the step having an average density closest to but not less than:
___ a. 1.00
___ b. 1.10
___ c. 1.20
___ d. 1.50

56. When establishing processor QC operating levels, the high density is determined by selecting the step having an average density closest to:
___ a. 3.00
___ b. 2.70
___ c. 2.20
___ d. 2.00

57. Recommended performance criteria for the analysis of mammography processing control charts call for MD and DD to be within ± ___ for no action to be taken.
___ a. 0.10
___ b. 0.01
___ c. 0.15
___ d. 0.50

58. A crossover should be performed whenever:
___ a. a new box of film is opened
___ b. developer is replaced with unseasoned chemistry

____ c. establishing operating values for processor QC

____ d. more than one but not all of the above

59. The device used to confirm that the generator is producing the kVp as indicated on the control panel is a:

____ a. step wedge

____ b. copper step meter

____ c. R-meter

____ d. digital kVp meter

60. When performing an exposure-time accuracy test with a digital x-ray timer, it is important to do a minimum of ____ exposures for each selected time station.

____ a. 2

____ b. 3

____ c. 5

____ d. no minimum is required

61. The mammographic phantom used for QC tests should be approximately equivalent to a 4.2 cm thick compressed breast consisting of what percentage of glandular tissue?

____ a. 10

____ b. 30

____ c. 50

____ d. 60

62. Mammographic phantom images should have a background density measurement never less than:

____ a. 1.0 ±0.1

____ b. 1.0 ±0.2

____ c. 1.2 ±0.2

____ d. 1.2 ±0.1

63. What equipment is needed when performing an AEC backup time test?

____ a. AEC test phantom and stopwatch

____ b. lead apron and stopwatch

____ c. lead apron and AEC test phantom

____ d. densitometer and AEC test phantom

64. Film illuminators used to view radiographs should have a brightness level of:
    ____ a. 1500 nit
    ____ b. 1200 nit
    ____ c. 1000 nit
    ____ d. 800 nit

65. The ACR requires that both the sensitometer and densitometer be recalibrated every:
    ____ a. year
    ____ b. 18 months
    ____ c. 2 years
    ____ d. none of the above are correct

66. Star test patterns are used to measure:
    ____ a. film resolution
    ____ b. filament bloom
    ____ c. focal spot size
    ____ d. linearity

67. When performing a test to confirm that the small and large focal spots are within the tube manufacturer's stated specifications, the test instrument should be placed:
    ____ a. on the faceplate of the collimator
    ____ b. on the image receptor
    ____ c. on the radiographic table
    ____ d. more than one but not all are acceptable

68. The most important QC area in the overall quality assurance program is the:
    ____ a. darkroom
    ____ b. record-keeping process
    ____ c. collection and analysis of data
    ____ d. medical physicist's assessment

69. What tools are required for processor monitoring?
    I. thermometer
    II. sensitometer
    III. densitometer
    IV. QC film
    ____ a. II and III
    ____ b. I, II, and III
    ____ c. II, III, and IV
    ____ d. I, II, III, and IV

70. Processor control strips should be kept as part of the permanent record for at least:
_____ a. 6 months
_____ b. 12 months
_____ c. 18 months
_____ d. 24 months

71. When testing with a digital kVp for kVp accuracy at the 70, 90, and 100 kVp stations meter, you obtained 68 kVp, 94 kVp, and 100 kVp. Are the kVp values within acceptable parameters?
_____ a. yes
_____ b. no
_____ c. more information needed

72. How often should the fluoroscopic exposure reproducibility be checked?
_____ a. weekly
_____ b. monthly
_____ c. semiannually
_____ d. annually

73. When testing with a digital kVp meter for fluoroscopic kilovoltage accuracy at 80, 90, and 100 kV, you obtained 85 kVp, 94 kVp, and 100 kVp. Are the kVp values within acceptable parameters?
_____ a. yes
_____ b. no
_____ c. more information needed

74. In the manual fluoroscopic exposure mode, the maximum exposure rate should be ≤ _____ mC/kg/min.
_____ a. 0.10
_____ b. 1.0
_____ c. 1.3
_____ d. 1.5

75. In the automatic fluoroscopic exposure mode, the maximum exposure rate should be ≤ _____ R/min.
_____ a. 5
_____ b. 2.5
_____ c. 15
_____ d. 10

76. What holes should be clearly visualized with the low-contrast fluoroscopic test?
    ___ a. 1/4 and 3/16 inch
    ___ b. 1/8 and 3/16 inch
    ___ c. 1/8 and 1/4 inch
    ___ d. 1/16 and 1/8 inch

77. The low-contrast fluoroscopic test should be performed for the:
    I. TV monitor
    II. Spot film device
    III. Linearity
    ___ a. I only
    ___ b. II only
    ___ c. I and II
    ___ d. I, II, and III

78. Which of the following recognizes variation over a period of time and encourages evaluation of the pattern of variation so that actions toward betterment can be initiated?
    ___ a. QC
    ___ b. QA
    ___ c. QI
    ___ d. all of the above

79. Choose the nonstatistical tool used to generate a large volume of ideas for the list below:
    ___ a. flowchart
    ___ b. matrix
    ___ c. brainstorming
    ___ d. more than one but not all of the above

80. This chart is used to monitor one or more processes over time to determine if there are shifts or trends:
    ___ a. flowchart
    ___ b. run chart
    ___ c. Pareto chart
    ___ d. central tendency chart

81. A QI team brainstormed to identify factors that produced variability in a process. Team members categorized these variables as to equipment, process, manpower, materials, and methods. What tool would they use to visually display the results of the brainstorming session?
    _____ a. flowchart
    _____ b. Pareto chart
    _____ c. cause and effect diagram
    _____ d. control chart

82. For the following data, calculate the median:
    14, 9, 36, 3, 98, 105, 18
    _____ a. 18
    _____ b. 27
    _____ c. 40
    _____ d. 50

83. If the causes of variation in a process are constant, then measuring the outcomes will produce a set of data points that have a predictable spread that can be mathematically modeled. This spread is called the:
    _____ a. average
    _____ b. mode
    _____ c. standard deviation
    _____ d. skew

84. FOCUS-PDCA is an organized problem-solving process that yields an avenue for continuous improvement. What does the C in FOCUS represent?
    _____ a. causes for process variation are identified
    _____ b. clarify the problem and current knowledge of the process
    _____ c. collect data
    _____ d. none of the above

85. Which of the following methods is used to narrow down options without discouraging specific team members who espouse various hypotheses?
    _____ a. checksheets
    _____ b. multivoting
    _____ c. regression analysis
    _____ d. more than one but not all of the above

86. Control charts are popular forms of presentation items for quality improvement teams. Upper and lower control limits for these charts are typically set at sigma. What is another name for this term?
    ____ a. standard deviation
    ____ b. coefficient of variation
    ____ c. spread
    ____ d. highest and lowest range

87. An alternative to the FOCUS-PDCA model is the:
    ____ a. seven-step model
    ____ b. statistical tools model
    ____ c. Deming's principles
    ____ d. more than one but not all of the above

88. This analysis tool is designed to determine whether there is a relationship between two variables. It can be used to examine the relationship between a key quality characteristic and potential process variables. What is this tool?
    ____ a. storyboard
    ____ b. scatter plot
    ____ c. Pareto chart
    ____ d. cause and effect diagram

89. The symbolic representation of standard deviation is:
    ____ a. σ
    ____ b. s
    ____ c. sd
    ____ d. $s\sigma$

90. A bar graph describing a monitored event in descending order from left to right is termed a:
    ____ a. Pareto chart
    ____ b. histogram
    ____ c. matrix
    ____ d. distribution chart

91. What is the standard deviation for the following set of numbers?

    2, 8, 22, 36, 50, and 72
    ____ a. 31.7
    ____ b. 29
    ____ c. 25
    ____ d. 24.2

92. The ΣX of a group of numbers is 480. The n equals 14. What is the mean?

_____ a. 34.29
_____ b. 17.14
_____ c. 68.57
_____ d. more information is needed

93. This tool represents the easiest and fastest method for documenting information about a process.

_____ a. pie chart
_____ b. check sheet
_____ c. run chart
_____ d. matrix

94. Which of the following measures is **not** a statistical tool?

_____ a. frequency distributions
_____ b. central tendency
_____ c. spread
_____ d. survey

95. In the evaluation of a run chart, seven or more consecutive points above or below the center line indicates a _____ exists.

_____ a. trend
_____ b. controlled process
_____ c. shift
_____ d. pattern

96. What is the one sigma rule?

_____ a. occurs when eight or more consecutive points are within one standard deviation from the center line
_____ b. occurs when four or five consecutive points are one standard deviation on the same side as the center line
_____ c. occurs when two or three consecutive points are one standard deviation on the same side as the center line
_____ d. none of the above

97. Health status and disability represent:

_____ a. a structure
_____ b. a process
_____ c. an outcome
_____ d. a concept

98. A central aspect for applying quality improvement relies on identifying and monitoring:
    ____ a. outcome indicators
    ____ b. process limitations
    ____ c. system components
    ____ d. none of the above

99. Choose an example of an indicator from the following list:
    ____ a. infection rates
    ____ b. timeliness of diagnostic test
    ____ c. accuracy of payroll
    ____ d. all of the above are indicators

100. When beginning a quality improvement project, it is only after the process in question is understood that data about process variables can be collected to determine if the process is in control. Which of the following tools is used to gain an understanding of the process?
    ____ a. run chart
    ____ b. flowchart
    ____ c. both a and b
    ____ d. none of the above

101. This tool presents measurements in a way that displays the nature of the distribution. The chart represents the frequency distribution of a set of data. What is this tool?
    ____ a. histogram
    ____ b. pie chart
    ____ c. run chart
    ____ d. control chart

102. From the list below, choose a model of data analysis.
    ____ a. research
    ____ b. benchmarking
    ____ c. both a and b
    ____ d. neither a nor b

103. When assessing patient satisfaction, data may include:
    ____ a. surveys of current patients
    ____ b. telephone response time
    ____ c. waiting time studies
    ____ d. a, b, and c are correct

104. A process is defined as:

_____ a. a defined set of causes and conditions that transforms inputs into outputs

_____ b. components of inputs only

_____ c. actions which produce outputs

_____ d. none of the above

105. What is another name for an Ishikawa diagram?

_____ a. flowchart

_____ b. cause control diagram

_____ c. fishbone diagram

_____ d. none of the above

106. In the analysis of a run chart, at least _____ points are needed to be valid.

_____ a. 35

_____ b. 10

_____ c. 20

_____ d. 25

107. A method of displaying the data, analyses, conclusions, and decisions made during the phases of a process improvement project is termed a:

_____ a. project notebook

_____ b. process accounting

_____ c. storyboard

_____ d. story notebook

108. The x-ray tube of a mobile fluoroscopic C-arm unit should maintain a SOD of:

_____ a. ≤ 15 inches

_____ b. ≤ 12 inches

_____ c. ≥ 15 inches

_____ d. ≥ 12 inches

109. What is the mode of the following group of numbers?

4, 10, 33, 51, 3, 17, 55, 3, 21, 92

_____ a. 3

_____ b. 19

_____ c. 29

_____ d. 92

110. Which of the following statements is true?

_____ a. upper and lower limits are not part of a run chart

_____ b. a run chart is used to map a process

_____ c. the center line of a run chart represents the median

_____ d. another name for a run chart is a shift chart

111. What tool does this figure represent?

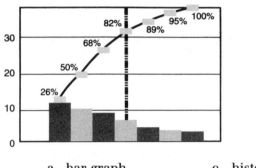

_____ a. bar graph   _____ c. histogram

_____ b. Pareto chart   _____ d. none of the above

112. In the following data set, what does N represent?

$$X = 45 \qquad\qquad N = 16 \qquad\qquad \sigma = 12.3$$

_____ a. raw score or number

_____ b. mean

_____ c. sample size

_____ d. coefficient of variation

113. What is the coefficient of variation for five exposures using the following exposure factors? The exposures conveyed mR readings of 210, 235, 221, 212, and 208. 100 mA @ 0.1 sec and 80 kVp.

_____ a. 0.0469

_____ b. 0.178

_____ c. 27

_____ d. 33.7

114. A method used to reduce the possibility of skewing during sample selection is:

_____ a. selection of a large sample ≥ 25

_____ b. randomization

_____ c. selection of a diverse sample

_____ d. none of the above

115. Frequency distributions depict data by how often an event or situation occurs.
    _____ a. true
    _____ b. false

116. When analyzing data dispersion, the percentiles often used are:
    _____ a. 15, 25, 75
    _____ b. 25, 75, 95
    _____ c. 25, 50, 75
    _____ d. 50, 75, 95

117. In the analysis of artifacts, lines that are parallel to the direction of film travel are most often caused by:
    _____ a. crossovers
    _____ b. guide shoes
    _____ c. entrance rollers
    _____ d. more than one but not all of the above

118. In the analysis of artifacts, artifacts with evenly spaced intervals of 1 inch are most often caused by:
    _____ a. crossovers
    _____ b. guide shoes
    _____ c. entrance rollers
    _____ d. more than one but not all of the above

119. In the analysis of artifacts, plus-density bands 1/8 inch wide are most often caused by:
    _____ a. crossovers
    _____ b. guide shoes
    _____ c. entrance rollers
    _____ d. more than one but not all of the above

120. Common perpendicular processing artifacts are referred to as:
    _____ a. pi lines
    _____ b. roller marks
    _____ c. streaks
    _____ d. stub lines

121. NCRP Report #99 states that the fluoroscopic image should not be less than _____ centimeter _____ than the specified diameter.
    _____ a. 1, smaller
    _____ b. 1, larger
    _____ c. 0.5, smaller
    _____ d. 0.5, larger

122. NCRP Report #99 states that fluoroscopic beam limitation be no greater than ____ of the SID at any tower height.
    ____ a. 12%
    ____ b. 10%
    ____ c. 5%
    ____ d. 3%

123. NCRP Report #99 states that the difference between the fluoroscopic image and the spot film image be no greater than ____ of the SID.
    ____ a. 12%
    ____ b. 10%
    ____ c. 5%
    ____ d. 3%

124. NCRP Report #99 states that the minimum HVL at 90 kVp is ____ mm AL.
    ____ a. 2.3
    ____ b. 2.5
    ____ c. 2.7
    ____ d. 3.0

125. The annual occupational exposure recommended by the NCRP is:
    ____ a. 50 mSv
    ____ b. 5000 mrem
    ____ c. 10 mSv
    ____ d. more than one but not all of the above

126. The annual effective dose for children under the age of 18 years recommended by the NCRP is:
    ____ a. 1 mSv
    ____ b. 5 mSv
    ____ c. 10 mSv
    ____ d. none of the above

127. The total effective dose for the embryo-fetus recommended by the NCRP is:
    ____ a. 0.5 mSv
    ____ b. 5 mSv
    ____ c. 10 mSv
    ____ d. 50 mrem

128. Report #99 by the NCRP states that the exposure reproducibility variance for an AEC device should be ± ____.

____ a. 12%
____ b. 10%
____ c. 5%
____ d. 3%

129. Which of the following is **not** a required QC test to be performed by the radiologic technologists?

____ a. radiation output rate
____ b. analysis of fixer retention in film
____ c. screen-film contact
____ d. phantom images

130. Visual checks of the equipment should be performed:

____ a. daily
____ b. weekly
____ c. monthly
____ d. annually

131. The mammography technologist should evaluate darkroom fog:

____ a. daily
____ b. weekly
____ c. semiannually
____ d. annually

132. The recommended performance criteria for fixer temperature for processing mammographic film is:

____ a. ± 3° F of the developer temperature
____ b. ± 5° F of the developer temperature
____ c. ± 2° C of the developer temperature
____ d. ± 5° C of the developer temperature

133. The recommended performance criteria for mammographic compression device performance is that a force of at least ____ pounds shall be provided.

____ a. 10
____ b. 15
____ c. 25
____ d. 45

134. When analyzing fixer retention in mammographic film, residual fixer should be less than:

_____ a. 5 micrograms per square centimeter

_____ b. 2 micrograms per square centimeter

_____ c. 0.5 micrograms per square centimeter

_____ d. 0.05 micrograms per square centimeter

135. OSHA recommends that a worker with occupational risk to _____ should be vaccinated.

_____ a. HBV

_____ b. HIV

_____ c. ACI

_____ d. more than one but not all of the above

136. A worker at risk for contracting a bloodborne pathogen should practice:

_____ a. universal precautions

_____ b. blood and body fluid precautions

_____ c. body substance isolation

_____ d. more than one but not all of the above

137. When referring to an MSDS, the term chemical means any:

_____ a. chemical compound

_____ b. mixture of elements

_____ c. mixture of compounds

_____ d. all of the above

138. Employers shall develop, implement, and maintain at each workplace, a/an _____ that includes policies for labeling and other forms of warning, material safety data sheets, and employee information and training.

_____ a. written hazard communication program

_____ b. department safety program

_____ c. infection control program

_____ d. department policy manual

139. The Safe Medical Device Act of 1990 requires that medical device users report to the ____ incidents that reasonably suggest that there is a probability that a medical device has caused or contributed to the death of a patient, serious injury or illness or a patient.

____ a. manufacturer
____ b. F.D.A.
____ c. both a and b are correct
____ d. none of the above

140. Serious illness or injury as defined by the Safe Medical Device Act of 1990 is an illness or injury that:

____ a. is life threatening
____ b. results in permanent impairment of bodily function
____ c. necessitates immediate medical or surgical intervention to preclude permanent impairment of a bodily function
____ d. a, b, and c are correct

ANSWERS TO MULTIPLE-CHOICE QUESTIONS

1. c. characteristic

2. a. increases, increases

3. a. luminesce

4. d. space charge

5. b. off-focus radiation

6. d. protective layer

7. a. screen efficiency

8. d. more than one but not all of the above

9. b. silver halide and gelatin

10. c. silver halide crystals

11. a. cracking artifacts

12. d. glutaraldehyde

13. a. brown films

14. d. specific gravity

15. c. both a and b

16. a. bromide

17. c. effective use of people

18. a. dryer exhaust

19. a. chemical oxidation

20. a. annually

21. b. faulty rectification

22. b. semiannually

23. b. .96 inches

24. c. 4 kVp

25. c. 10%

26. c. 13.44 mR/mAs

27. a. annually

28. b. no

29. c. half-value layer

30. b. acceptance testing, routine performance monitoring, and maintenance

31. a. is not producing artifacts

32. b. center, decreasing

33. a. annually

34. d. 1.2 inches

35. b. semiannually

36. d. 40 mesh/inch at the center of the image and 35 mesh/inch at the edge

37. a. daily

38. b. 2

39. c. semiannually

40. b. ±0.15

41. b. 30 to 50%

42. d. more than one but not all of the above

43. a. 2 to 3 m

44. a. 10%

45. b. step wedge

46. a. check developer thermostat setting

47. b. 18 months

48. d. annually

49. d. more than one but not all of the above

50. a. speed

51. b. quarterly

52. d. 0.5°F

53. a. 21

54. b. weekly

55. c. 1.20

56. c. 2.20

57. a. 0.10

58. a. a new box of film is opened

59. d. digital kVp meter

60. c. 5

61. c. 50

62. c. 1.2 ±0.2

63. b. lead apron and stopwatch

64. a. 1500 nit
65. b. 18 months
66. c. focal spot size
67. a. on the faceplate of the collimator
68. a. darkroom
69. d. I, II, III, and IV
70. b. 12 months
71. a. yes
72. c. semiannually
73. a. yes
74. c. 1.3
75. d. 10
76. a. 1/4 and 3/16 inch
77. c. I and II
78. c. QI
79. c. brainstorming
80. b. run chart
81. c. cause and effect diagram
82. a. 18
83. c. standard deviation
84. b. clarify the problem and current knowledge of the process
85. b. multivoting
86. a. standard deviation
87. a. seven-step model
88. b. scatter plot
89. a. σ
90. a. Pareto chart
91. d. 24.2
92. a. 34.29
93. b. check sheet
94. d. survey
95. c. shift

96. b. occurs when four or five consecutive points are one standard deviation on the same side as the center line

97. c. an outcome

98. a. outcome indicators

99. d. all of the above are indicators

100. b. flowchart

101. a. histogram

102. c. both a and b

103. d. a, b, and c are correct

104. a. a defined set of causes and conditions that transforms inputs into outputs

105. c. fishbone diagram

106. d. 25

107. c. storyboard

108. c. ≥ 15 inches

109. a. 3

110. a. upper and lower limits are not part of a run chart

111. b. Pareto chart

112. c. sample size

113. a. 0.0469

114. b. randomization

115. a. true

116. c. 25, 50, 75

117. b. guide shoes

118. b. guide shoes

119. c. entrance rollers

120. a. pi lines

121. a. 1, smaller

122. d. 3%

123. d. 3%

124. b. 2.5

125. d. more than one but not all of the above

126. a. 1 mSv

127. b. 5 mSv

128. c. 5%

129. a. radiation output rate

130. c. monthly

131. c. semiannually

132. b. ± 5° F of the developer temperature

133. c. 25

134. a. 5 micrograms per square centimeter

135. a. HBV

136. d. more than one but not all of the above

137. d. all of the above

138. a. written hazard communication program

139. c. both a and b are correct

140. d. a, b, and c are correct